OXFORD MEDICAL PUBLICATIONS

Fetal Cardiology

Oxford Specialist Handbooks published and forthcoming

General Oxford Specialist Handbooks
A Resuscitation Room Guide
Addiction Medicine
Day Case Surgery
Parkinson's Disease and Other Movement Disorders 2e
Perioperative Medicine, 2e
Pharmaceutical Medicine
Postoperative Complications, 2e
Renal Transplantation
Retrieval Medicine

Oxford Specialist Handbooks in Anaesthesia
Anaesthesia for Medical and Surgical Emergencies
Cardiac Anaesthesia
Neuroanaesthesia
Obstetric Anaesthesia
Ophthalmic Anaesthesia
Paediatric Anaesthesia
Regional Anaesthesia, Stimulation and Ultrasound Techniques
Thoracic Anaesthesia

Oxford Specialist Handbooks in Cardiology
Adult Congenital Heart Disease
Cardiac Catheterization and Coronary Intervention
Cardiac Electrophysiology and Catheter Ablation
Cardiovascular Computed Tomography
Cardiovascular Magnetic Resonance
Echocardiography, 2e
Fetal Cardiology
Heart Failure, 2e
Hypertension
Inherited Cardiac Disease
Nuclear Cardiology
Pacemakers and ICDs
Pulmonary Hypertension
Valvular Heart Disease

Oxford Specialist Handbooks in Critical Care
Advanced Respiratory Critical Care
Cardiothoracic Critical Care

Oxford Specialist Handbooks in End of Life Care
End of Life Care in Cardiology
End of Life Care in Dementia
End of Life Care in Nephrology
End of Life Care in Respiratory Disease
End of Life in the Intensive Care Unit

Oxford Specialist Handbooks in Infectious Disease
Infectious Disease Epidemiology
Manual of Childhood Infections 4e

Oxford Specialist Handbooks in Neurology
Epilepsy
Parkinson's Disease and Other Movement Disorders, 2e
Stroke Medicine, 2e

Oxford Specialist Handbooks in Oncology
Practical Management of Complex Cancer Pain

Oxford Specialist Handbooks in Paediatrics
Paediatric Dermatology
Paediatric Endocrinology and Diabetes
Paediatric Gastroenterology, Hepatology, and Nutrition
Paediatric Haematology and Oncology
Paediatric Intensive Care
Paediatric Nephrology, 2e
Paediatric Neurology, 2e
Paediatric Palliative Medicine, 2e
Paediatric Radiology
Paediatric Respiratory Medicine
Paediatric Rheumatology

Oxford Specialist Handbooks in Pain Medicine
Spinal Interventions in Pain Management

Oxford Specialist Handbooks in Psychiatry
Addiction Medicine, 2e
Child and Adolescent Psychiatry
Forensic Psychiatry
Medical Psychotherapy
Old Age Psychiatry

Oxford Specialist Handbooks in Radiology
Interventional Radiology
Musculoskeletal Imaging
Pulmonary Imaging
Thoracic Imaging

Oxford Specialist Handbooks in Surgery
Cardiothoracic Surgery, 2e
Colorectal Surgery
Gastric and Oesophageal Surgery
Hand Surgery
Hepatopancreatobiliary Surgery
Neurosurgery
Operative Surgery, 2e
Oral and Maxillofacial Surgery, 2e
Otolaryngology and Head and Neck Surgery
Paediatric Surgery
Plastic and Reconstructive Surgery
Surgical Oncology
Urological Surgery
Vascular Surgery, 2e

Oxford Specialist Handbooks in Cardiology

Fetal Cardiology

Second edition

Dr Nick Archer

Paediatric Cardiologist (retired)
Oxford University Hospitals

and

Former Honorary Clinical Senior Lecturer
University of Oxford, UK

Dr Nicky Manning

Fetal Cardiologist
Great Ormond Street Hospital, London

and

Oxford University Hospitals, UK

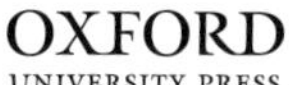

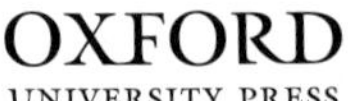

Great Clarendon Street, Oxford, OX2 6DP,
United Kingdom

Oxford University Press is a department of the University of Oxford. It furthers the University's objective of excellence in research, scholarship, and education by publishing worldwide. Oxford is a registered trade mark of Oxford University Press in the UK and in certain other countries

Impression: 1

Published in the United States of America by Oxford University Press
198 Madison Avenue, New York, NY 10016, United States of America

British Library Cataloguing in Publication Data
Data available

Library of Congress Control Number: 2018931184

ISBN 978–0–19–876652–0 (pbk.)

Printed and bound in China by
C&C Offset Printing Co., Ltd.

Forewords to the first edition

At the heart of fetal medicine and obstetrics, fetal cardiology plays a crucial part in our understanding and observation of fetal disease, as well as in our knowledge about congenital heart disease. Increasing numbers of adults have congenital heart disease and yet there is little available that describes the development, prenatal diagnosis, and treatments available in a concise format. With huge practical experience of the subject, the authors, as experts in prenatal diagnosis, monitoring and treatment, and in childhood management of disease, are amply qualified to write what is an amazing little book that covers this subject in a clear, concise but comprehensive manner.

Lawrence Impey
Consultant in Obstetrics and Fetal Medicine
The John Radcliffe Hospital
Oxford
2009

Fetal cardiology is a young clinical specialty which was made possible by the development of high-resolution ultrasound. At its inception in the early 1980s, the expectation was that structural heart defects would most likely be detected by detailed scanning of the fetal heart in those pregnancies designated to be at high risk for the presence of fetal cardiac abnormality. However, it soon became apparent that most fetal heart defects were, in fact, detected because a heart abnormality was suspected at routine midtrimester anomaly scanning in pregnancies not deemed to be high risk. This meant that, from its early days, fetal cardiology has been a cooperative venture shared principally between obstetric ultrasonographers, fetal medicine practitioners and subspecialist paediatric cardiologists.

It is therefore both symbolic and appropriate that this handbook is co-authored by specialists in fetal medicine and paediatric cardiology respectively. Their combined perspective is apparent in the broad-based and logical approach to the subject, which reflects a 'real life' practical experience not just of fetal cardiac diagnosis, but crucially also of the wider clinical assessment which is so important in counselling. This book will benefit a broad readership, especially sonographers, nurses, and physicians involved variously in fetal medicine, obstetrics, paediatric cardiology or adult congenital heart disease.

It may also be considered testament to the rapid growth in practice, knowledge, and importance of such a young specialty that this timely 'handbook', despite being concise and clinical in content, runs to over 300 merited pages!

Ian Sullivan
Consultant Cardiologist
Great Ormond Street Hospital for Children
London
2009

Forewords to the second edition

Fetal cardiology is relevant to obstetrics as well as paediatrics. Antenatal detection rates of congenital heart disease are increasing. The role that the heart may play in the diagnosis and monitoring of fetal disease, such as growth restriction is also increasing. This little book has established itself as invaluable to all who encounter the field of fetal cardiology. It was written, and now updated, by two experts with huge practical experience of screening, diagnosis, monitoring and treatment, including *in utero*, postnatally and in childhood. It offers an excellent introduction to fetal cardiology and should be essential reading for doctors in fetal medicine and sonographers.

Lawrence Impey
Consultant in Obstetrics and Fetal Medicine
Oxford University Hospital
2018

It is testimony to the increasingly important role of fetal cardiology that a timely second edition of this handbook is now available. The new edition follows the user friendly format of the original. The main emphasis remains the recognition and assessment of structural heart defects, but there is also extensive coverage of cardiac aspects of wider fetal medicine concern. Arguably, the most important development in medicine over the past decade has been the increasingly sophisticated identification of genetic determinants of development and disease. This edition contains appropriately expanded description of contemporary prenatal genetic assessment relevant to clinical fetal cardiology. Advanced fetal cardiac imaging techniques are also included, although it is continuing computer development giving rise to steady improvement in the high resolution of "conventional" ultrasound which continues to give the most insight into subtleties of fetal cardiac physiology. In summary, this welcome new edition successfully updates a succinct source of the core information required to support and guide multidisciplinary fetal cardiology practitioners.

Ian Sullivan
Consultant in Paediatric and Fetal Cardiology (retired)
Great Ormond Street Hospital for Children
London
2018

Preface to the first edition

In two decades, fetal cardiology has developed from the ability to recognize normal and abnormal fetal cardiac structure by ultrasound to a specialty in its own right. Ultrasound is still at the centre of diagnosis and management to the extent that all practitioners have to be conversant with it and at least competent in its use. The nature of the specialty means that professionals from many different backgrounds are involved and are required to have some knowledge in areas which are not their primary specialty. Fetal cardiology now involves so much more than just confirming normality or diagnosing structural abnormality of the fetal heart. The aim of this handbook is to bring together sufficient information in an accessible single source to allow professionals from many different disciplines to have a sound understanding of the scope and limitations of fetal cardiac diagnosis and treatment. We hope that this book will be of practical clinical value to all involved in fetal cardiac assessment or in the management of feto-maternal problems.

Nick Archer
Nicky Manning
Oxford 2009

Preface to the second edition

Even in the year 2018, ultrasound is still the standard method for defining fetal cardiac anatomy and function, and diagnostic expectations and accuracy continue to rise. This is why we have replaced the majority of the images from the first edition.

However, there is more to assessment of the fetal cardiovascular system than echocardiography alone and we hope that this new edition again illustrates this important point.

We are grateful to our colleagues from supporting specialities for their valuable input to our book, both from their specific clinical contribution but also their unfailing enthusiasm and encouragement without which we would still be writing.

In particular, we would like to thank Dr Deirdre Cilliers (Consultant Geneticist, Oxford), Dr David Black (Consultant Fetal and Paediatric Cardiologist, Southampton and Oxford), Dr Alex Jones (Consultant Paediatric Cardiologist, Oxford), and Dr David Lloyd (Clinical Research Fellow, Evelina Children's Hospital, London), not only for broadening our horizons but also for their valuable written contributions to some chapters.

As with the first edition, we hope that this book will serve as an accessible source of knowledge and clinical guidance to enable professionals from different backgrounds to appreciate the scope and limitations of fetal cardiology and to incorporate it appropriately into their clinical work.

Nick Archer
Nicky Manning
Oxford 2018

Contents

Symbols and abbreviations

➲	cross reference
🖱	website
2D	2-dimensional
3D	3-dimensional
4D	4-dimensional
A	anterior
ACE	angiotensin-converting enzyme
AET	atrial ectopic tachycardia
Ao	aorta
APV	absent pulmonary valve
AS	aortic stenosis
ASD	atrial septal defect
AV	atrioventricular
AVNRT	atrioventricular nodal re-entry tachycardia
AVRT	atrioventricular re-entry tachycardia
AVSD	atrioventricular septal defect
bpm	beats per minute
CAUD	caudal
cAVSD	complete atrioventricular septal defect
CEPH	cephalad
cffDNA	cell-free fetal DNA
CGA	comparative genomic hybridization
CHB	compete heart block
CHD	congenital heart disease
C:T	cardiac:thoracic (ratio)
CTG	cardiotocograph
CVS	chorionic villus sampling
CW	continuous wave
DA	ductus arteriosus
DC	dichorionic
DCM	dilated cardiomyopathy
DORV	double outlet right ventricle
DZ	dizygotic
ECG	electrocardiogram
FISH	fluorescence *in situ* hybridization
HCM	hypertrophic cardiomyopathy
HLHS	hypoplastic left heart syndrome
IVC	inferior vena cava
IVS	interventricular septum
JET	junctional ectopic tachycardia
LA	left atrium

LQTS	long QT syndrome
LV	left ventricle/ventricular
LVOT	left ventricular outflow tract
m/sec	metres per second
MAPCA	major aortopulmonary collateral artery
min	minute(s)
MC	monochorionic
MPLA	multiplex ligation-dependent probe amplification
MRI	magnetic resonance imaging
MV	mitral valve
MZ	monozygotic
NSAID	non-steroidal anti-inflammatory drug
NT	nuchal translucency
P	posterior
PA	pulmonary artery
PAC	premature atrial contraction
PAIVS	pulmonary atresia with intact ventricular septum
pAVSD	partial atrioventricular septal defect
PCR	polymerase chain reaction
PI	pulsatility index
PJRT	permanent junctional reciprocating tachycardia
PS	pulmonary stenosis
PV	pulmonary valve
PW	pulsed wave
QTc	corrected QT interval
R	right
RA	right atrium
RV	right ventricle
RVOT	right ventricular outflow tract
sec	second(s)
Sp	spine
SR	sinus rhythm
SSRI	selective serotonin re-uptake inhibitor
St	stomach
STIC	spatiotemporal image correlation
SVC	superior vena cava
SVE	supraventricular ectopic
SVT	supraventricular tachycardia
TAPVD	total anomalous pulmonary venous drainage
TGA	transposition of the great arteries
TR	tricuspid regurgitation
TTTS	twin–twin transfusion syndrome
TV	tricuspid valve
U/S	ultrasound
VSD	ventricular septal defect

Chapter 1

Introduction

Role of fetal cardiology

Fetal cardiology contributes to many areas of fetal care including:

- Diagnosis and management of fetal cardiac disease:
  - This is now an integral part of fetal assessment and therefore incorporates prenatal diagnosis, fetomaternal medicine, genetics, neonatology, paediatric cardiology, and cardiac surgery.
- A fetal cardiac service must have close interaction with these other specialties, ideally being sited on the same campus.
- Communication between practitioners in these different specialties as well as with the families involved is key to delivering optimum management.
- It is important that professionals of many disciplines understand the scope and the limitations of what fetal cardiac assessment has to offer.

Scope of fetal cardiology

The following roles are part of fetal cardiac care:

- Screening is normally performed by sonographers or obstetricians but fetal cardiologists need to be involved in training, updating, and maintaining their skills.
- Diagnosis or exclusion of structural congenital heart disease (CHD) in those considered at increased risk.
- Assessment and management of fetal arrhythmias.
- Assessment of functional heart disease in many settings.
- Cardiac assessment may contribute importantly to possible syndrome evaluation.
- Counselling in detail about the cardiac diagnosis and its fetal and postnatal implications is an integral part of detailed cardiac assessment.
- Allowing informed decision-making in terms of invasive testing ± continuation of the pregnancy.
- Planning pregnancy management, and occasionally intervention.
- Planning delivery details.
- Alerting those involved in neonatal management.
- Preparing a postnatal plan.
- Helping in discussions about recurrence risk.

Limitations of fetal cardiology

Families and professionals need to be aware of the limitations of even an expert fetal cardiac evaluation:

- Time-consuming for patients and practitioners.
- Fetal echocardiographic diagnoses are not always right/complete.
- Image quality is influenced by:
  - maternal body mass index (BMI)
  - gestation
  - fetal position
  - number of fetuses
  - liquor volume.
- Some lesions are hard to diagnose and impossible to rule out eg: coarctation of the aorta, total anomalous pulmonary venous drainage (TAPVD), coronary abnormalities.
- It is not always possible to give a precise prognosis for lesions detected *in utero*.
- Normal variants and findings of uncertain significance cause unnecessary anxiety.

Chapter 2

Aetiology of fetal heart disease

Introduction

- The incidence of CHD is approximately 8:1000 live births, and is higher in the antenatal population.
- Aetiology:
  - environmental factors
  - a genetic predisposition
  - specific genetic causes are increasingly being identified.
- Epigenetic factors may modify the phenotypic cardiac manifestation.
- Approximately 40% of fetuses with CHD have additional non-cardiac anomalies:
  - structural
  - syndromic
  - chromosomal
  - abnormal microarray.
- Consanguinity is a risk factor for abnormalities including cardiac.
- Antenatal identification of aetiology allows accurate counselling.
- Counselling includes discussion of:
  - the cardiac lesion and its evolution, *in utero* and postnatally
  - the longer-term prognosis
  - risk of non-cardiac anomalies
  - the risk for recurrence in subsequent pregnancies.
- In spite of increasing knowledge in this area, for the majority of cases no specific cause can be identified.

Maternal factors

Any genetically determined abnormality in either parent clearly has a relevant risk to offspring. It is unclear as to whether or not other paternal factors are relevant.

Some maternal conditions are recognized to increase the risk for CHD in the fetus.

Diabetes mellitus

- Type 1 diabetes (pre-gestational diabetes) increases the risk of CHD to 3–5%:
  - Hyperglycaemia modifies proliferation and migration of neural crest cells.
  - Poor glycaemic control in the 1st trimester increases the risk for all anomalies including cardiac.
- The risk for type 2 diabetes, controlled with metformin between pregnancies, is harder to define and may also be determined by glycaemic control in early pregnancy:
  - If there is a need to start insulin in the 1st trimester, the risk for CHD might be similar to type 1 diabetes.
- Gestational diabetics, by definition, should have normal blood glucose levels in the 1st trimester, but higher levels later and therefore there is an increased risk for fetal CHD.
- Poor control during pregnancy for all diabetics increases the risk for fetal hyperinsulinism and macrosomia with associated hypertrophic cardiomyopathy which resolves spontaneously postnatally.
- Specific cardiac lesions seen in fetuses of diabetic mothers include:
  - ventricular septal defect (VSD)
  - transposition of the great arteries (TGA)
  - double outlet right ventricle (DORV)
  - heterotaxy
  - hypoplastic left heart syndrome
  - common arterial trunk.

Phenylketonuria

- Phenylketonuria (PKU) is an autosomal recessive single gene disorder causing high maternal levels of phenylalanine (which crosses the placenta and is teratogenic):
  - Associated with 10–15% increased risk of CHD if mother not on diet.
  - Also growth retardation and microcephaly.
- Cardiac lesions associated with PKU include:
  - tetralogy of Fallot
  - coarctation of the aorta
  - VSD
  - complex lesions.

Therapeutic maternal drug exposure

Maternal medications which cross the placenta are recognized to increase the risk for all structural anomalies including cardiac, and include:

- anticonvulsant therapy

- lithium
- angiotensin-converting enzyme (ACE) inhibitors
- antidepressants
- non-steroidal anti-inflammatory drug (NSAIDs)
- retinoic acid.

Anticonvulsant therapy

- The risk for CHD is probably not as high as previously thought, especially if high-dose folic acid has been taken prior to conception:
  - The risk of teratogenicity must be balanced against morbidity and mortality of seizures during (and after) pregnancy.
- The risk is higher in women requiring polytherapy.
- Risk for sodium valproate > phenytoin > carbamazepine > phenobarbitone and is probably dose related.
- Newer drugs, e.g. lamotrigine, probably do not increase the risk for CHD and therefore are the drugs of choice if appropriate.
- Cardiac lesions include:
  - VSD
  - atrial septal defect (ASD)
  - pulmonary stenosis (PS)
  - aortic stenosis (AS).

Lithium

- Historically considered high risk particularly for Ebstein's anomaly but recent studies have not confirmed this and the risk is now considered to be low.

ACE inhibitors

- ACE inhibitors are widely used for maternal hypertension but are discontinued in the 2nd and 3rd trimesters because of their association with fetopathy.
- Recent evidence suggests they could be teratogenic if used in 1st trimester, causing various anomalies including cardiac, perhaps by inducing fetal hypotension.

Antidepressants

- Selective serotonin re-uptake inhibitors (SSRIs) are widely used and appear safe with the possible exception of paroxetine which may be associated with an increased incidence of ASDs and VSDs.
- Studies give conflicting information and overall the increased risk, if present, is small and maternal well-being is a priority.

NSAIDs

- This group of drugs is used postnatally specifically to close the ductus arteriosus in premature babies in whom the duct has failed to close spontaneously.
- There is a risk that use of these drugs antenatally could cause premature closure of the duct *in utero* leading to serious consequences to haemodynamics including:
  - right heart failure
  - hydrops
  - complications for lung vasculature development.

- When this group of drugs is used prenatally for tocolysis, monitoring during the 1st week of use is essential:
  - Changes are reversible if the NSAID is stopped.
- Use of NSAIDs for maternal analgesia (which may be bought over the counter) carries a similar risk.

Retinoic acid

- A vitamin A derivative prescribed for acne.
- Widely recognized for its teratogenicity, including cardiac defects in the form of conotruncal and arch anomalies.
- Women are advised to use contraception for at least 1 month after finishing treatment.

Non-therapeutic drug exposure

- Risks for this category are hard to define, partly as information about quantity and timing of consumption may be incomplete.

Alcohol

- Alcohol consumption in early pregnancy is common and may be associated with an increased risk of CHD.
- High and prolonged alcohol intake is teratogenic and may result in the fetal alcohol syndrome with a combination of anomalies including cardiac.
- 'Binge drinking' in the 1st trimester presents the highest risk.
- Risk of CHD depends on intake and timing:
  - Up to 30% in cases of fetal alcohol syndrome.
  - Mainly for septal defects and tetralogy of Fallot.
- Ethanol probably interferes with protein synthesis.

Cocaine and marijuana

- Notoriously difficult to quantify and probably under-reported but the risk is generally considered to be increased.

Maternal infections

- Mothers reporting a febrile illness during the 1st trimester have a 2-fold increased risk of CHD, especially for obstructive lesions.

Rubella

- Maternal infection with rubella is associated with an increased risk of structural CHD, in addition to deafness and cataracts.
- 80% risk of congenital anomalies if acquired during the 1st trimester.
- Rubella vaccination is contraindicated during pregnancy as it may be associated with congenital anomalies.

Monochorionic twins

See ➔ Chapter 23.

Assisted reproduction

The risk is hard to define, especially as a significant number of these pregnancies will be multiple, with their own risk see ➔ Chapter 23.

Genetic factors

- Even in the absence of a recognizable genetic aetiology:
  - After one pregnancy with CHD, the risk for recurrence in a subsequent pregnancy rises from approximately 1% (8:1000) background risk to 2–3%.
  - For 2 previously affected children, the risk rises to 10%.
  - If a parent has CHD, the risk to their offspring is between 3% and 20%, depending on the cardiac lesion and is higher for maternal than paternal CHD.
  - In approximately 50% of recurrences the cardiac lesion will be the same as in the index case.
- Overall 30–40% of prenatally diagnosed CHD are associated with non-cardiac anomalies.

Genetic causes

The genome

- Each cell has 23 pairs of chromosomes:
  - 22 pairs of autosomes
  - 1 pair of sex chromosomes.
- One of each chromosome pair is inherited from each parent.
- These chromosomes carry about 21,000 genes.
- Genetic causes of CHD can be disorders of either:
  - chromosomes
  - single genes.
- Genetic causes of CHD may be either:
  - isolated cardiac abnormalities
  - include non-cardiac components (syndromes).
- Genetic disorders are commonly *de novo* or can be inherited from a parent.
- Inherited genetic conditions can show variable penetrance and thus not be clinically apparent in a parent even when present.
- If there is a known genetic condition in a family then prenatal genetic diagnosis may be possible.

Chromosomal disorders—syndromic

Numerical (aneuploidy)

- The human diploid chromosome complement is 46 and any change in this number is described as aneuploidy.
- The error usually arises as a result of non-disjunction at the time of cell division and can affect the autosomes (chromosomes 1–22) or the sex chromosomes (X and Y).
- All numerical chromosome anomalies have a strong association with CHD as well as other structural anomalies, many of which may be detected prenatally (see Table 2.1).
- In trisomies, there is an extra chromosome (46 + 1); in monosomies, there is loss of a chromosome (45).
- Aneuploidy is the most frequently prenatally encountered chromosome abnormality.
- Common aneuploidies are described in Table 2.1.

Structural

- This group includes chromosome microdeletions, duplications, translocations, and other rearrangements.
- Deletions are more commonly associated with CHD and the size of the deletion will determine whether it can be detected by microscopy or whether specific molecular cytogenetic techniques are required.
- Karyotyping (➲ Chapter 8) can detect larger deletions.
- Microarray (➲ Chapter 8) is the preferred test as it detects smaller changes.
- Fluorescence *in situ* hybridization (FISH, ➲ Chapter 8) can be used if looking for a specific chromosomal diagnosis such as 22q11 abnormalities.

Table 2.1 Commonly identified aneuploidies and associated cardiac lesions

Syndrome	Chromosome anomaly	Incidence (live births)	Frequency of cardiac lesions	Commonest cardiac lesions
Down syndrome	+21	*1:700	40–50%	Atrioventricular septal defect (AVSD) VSD ASD Tetralogy of Fallot
Patau syndrome	+13	*1:9500	80%	ASD VSD Complex lesions
Edward syndrome	+18	*1:6000	100%	VSD ASD DORV Valvar dysplasia
Turner syndrome	XO	1:2500	35%	Bicuspid aortic valve Coarctation Hypoplastic left heart

* Risk increases with advancing maternal age.

- Many deletions and duplications occur *de novo* and some of the cardiac diagnoses may not be detectable prenatally such as supravalvar aortic stenosis and pulmonary artery branch stenosis.
- If one family member is affected, definitive prenatal diagnosis may be possible.
- Structural chromosomal abnormalities so far defined include those listed in Table 2.2:
  - 22q11 deletion (Di George syndrome) is the commonest detected *in utero*.
  - 22q11 duplication is being increasingly detected with features not unlike 22q11 deletion.
  - Williams (Beuren) syndrome is rarely suspected antenatally.

Chromosomal disorders—non-syndromic

- Microduplications and deletions are increasingly found to be contributing to isolated heart malformations.
- Tetralogy of Fallot is commonly associated with these chromosomal variants.
- Many of these deletions and duplications may also be seen with syndromic disorders reflecting the variability of the phenotype.
- Non-penetrance or a syndromic phenotype may be present in other family members.
- Microarrays will identify these chromosomal disorders (➔ Chapter 8).
- These chromosomal disorders may be identified by whole genome sequencing, both as causal and as incidental findings.

Table 2.2 Examples of structural chromosomal abnormalities with CHD

Syndrome	Chromosomal anomaly	Frequency of cardiac lesions (live birth incidence)	Common cardiac malformations
1p36 deletion syndrome	1p36 deletion	40–70%	Many structural lesions, cardiomyopathy in childhood
Williams syndrome (1:10000)	7q11 deletion	>80% (1:10,000)	Supravalvar AS, supravalvar PS
Kleefstra syndrome	9q34 deletion	50%	ASD/VSD, tetralogy of Fallot, coarctation aorta, bicuspid aortic valve, PS
Jacobsen syndrome	11q23 deletion	56–70%	VSD, atrioventricular valve abnormalities, coarctation, hypoplastic left heart syndrome, complex lesions
DiGeorge syndrome	22q11 deletion	85%(1:4000)	Tetralogy, interrupted aortic arch, pulmonary atresia + VSD, common arterial trunk
Cat eye syndrome	22q11inv/dup	60–70%	TAPVD, ASD, PDA, tetralogy, complex lesions

Single gene disorders—syndromic

- There are many single gene disorders involved in syndromic CHD (see Table 2.3).
- These may follow autosomal dominant, autosomal recessive, or X-linked inheritance patterns.
- Penetrance and expression vary and many arise as *de novo* mutations.
- It may be possible to detect the condition prenatally if there is a confirmed mutation identified in a family member.
- Single gene tests (sequencing the DNA) are usually used to confirm the disorder suspected clinically in a patient.
- Increasingly, gene panel tests are used to test for single gene disorders, e.g. Noonan syndrome.
- In future, whole genome sequencing will become increasingly available to test for these disorders.
- Genotype–phenotype correlations occur in syndromic CHD conditions with multiple causative genes and this may help direct clinical management:
    - For example, PS occurs commonly in patients with Noonan syndrome caused by *PTPN11* or *SOS1* gene mutations, whereas *RAF1* or *RIT1* gene mutations are associated with a higher chance of cardiomyopathy.

Table 2.3 Examples of single gene syndromic disorders with CHD

Syndrome	Associated gene	Frequency of cardiac lesions	Most common cardiac malformations
CHARGE	*CHD7*	75–80%	Tetralogy of Fallot, AV canal defects, aortic arch anomalies
RASopathy disorders (commonest: Noonan syndrome)	Many genes, most common *PTPN11*	Noonan syndrome 80% Costello syndrome 45–60%,	PS, hypertrophic cardiomyopathy (Noonan and Leopard), arrhythmias (Costello) ASD,VSD
Alagille	*JAG1*	93%	PS, tetralogy of Fallot, PA, septal defects, complex
Holt–Oram	*TBX5*	75%	ASD, VSD, conduction defects
Ellis–van Creveld	*EVC*	50–60%	ASD, AVSD, persistent left superior vena cava
VACTERL	No known gene	75%	ASD, VSD, tetralogy of Fallot
Tuberous sclerosis (➔ Chapter 20)	*TSC 1* *TSC 2*	Approx. 50% of infants have cardiac tumours	Cardiac rhabdomyomata, usually multiple

- Confirming a diagnosis would also help determine the recurrence risk:
  - It may also allow prenatal testing or pre-implantation genetic diagnosis to be offered.
- Some of the more common single gene disorders with CHD are listed in Table 2.3

Single gene disorders—non-syndromic

- Non-syndromic CHD can be caused by a single gene disorder or by a multifactorial inheritance pattern.
- Many of the genes involved in isolated cardiac anomalies display incomplete or non-penetrance which can complicate diagnosis.
- Many of the genes that are involved in non-syndromic CHD are also involved in syndromic single gene disorders, demonstrating the variability of the phenotype.
- Consider investigating these genes where there are two or more 1st- or 2nd-degree family members with a congenital cardiac malformation.
- Cardiac gene panel tests or whole genome sequencing can be used to identify mutations although these mutations are still identified in relatively few patients.
- An example of a gene involved in non-syndromic CHD is the *NKX2.5* gene which usually causes autosomal dominant ASD and atrioventricular conduction defects but can cause lesions that are detectable in the fetus.

Risk of associated non-cardiac anomalies

- In clinical practice, it is either the fetal cardiac anomaly or a non-cardiac anomaly which starts the process of consideration of whether or not there is an underlying genetic cause.
- If a cardiac anomaly is identified, it is important to determine whether this is an 'isolated' finding or whether it is associated with other 'non-cardiac anomalies', structural, chromosomal, or syndromic.
- Some cardiac lesions have a stronger association with non-cardiac anomalies and vice versa, these are summarized in Boxes 2.1 and 2.2, and Table 2.4.

Box 2.1 Cardiac lesions with a lower association with non-cardiac anomalies

- Transposition of the great arteries
- Double inlet left ventricle
- Hypoplastic left heart syndrome
- Pulmonary atresia with intact septum
- Total anomalous pulmonary venous drainage
- Congenitally corrected transposition of the great arteries
- Ebstein anomaly.

Box 2.2 Cardiac lesions with a higher association with non-cardiac anomalies

- AVSD
- VSD
- Tetralogy of Fallot (including absent pulmonary valve syndrome)
- Pulmonary atresia with VSD
- Common arterial trunk
- Interrupted aortic arch
- Coarctation
- Dysplastic pulmonary valve.

Table 2.4 Associated non-cardiac anomalies for specific cardiac lesions

Cardiac lesion	Risk of non-cardiac anomaly	Commonest syndromes
AVSD	50%+	Trisomies 21,13, and 18 Various other syndromes
VSD	10–20% (depending on site)	Trisomies 21, 13, and 18 22q11 deletion syndrome Other structural anomalies
Tetralogy of Fallot, including absent pulmonary valve syndrome	6–20%	Trisomies 21, 13, and 18 22q11 deletion syndrome Alagille VACTERL CHARGE Other structural anomalies
Pulmonary atresia with VSD	25%+	22q11 deletion syndrome Alagille syndrome
Common arterial trunk	40%	22q11 deletion syndrome
Interrupted aortic arch	10–25%	22q11 deletion syndrome
Coarctation of the aorta	10%	Turner syndrome
Pulmonary valve dysplasia	50%+	Noonan syndrome

Prevention of congenital heart disease

- Primary prevention of CHD remains a challenge.
- Specific aetiologies may be avoidable:
  - Educating about risks of consanguinity.
  - Avoiding known teratogenic drugs.
  - Keeping rubella immunization rates high.
- Evidence suggests that high-dose folic acid reduces the risk for recurrence by up to 50%.
- Folate supplementation may also reduce severity of CHD.

Fetal origins of health and disease

- Mechanisms exist within the fetus which can influence organ development in response to altered resource availability.
- These factors may include:
  - changes in placental function
  - shared placental circulation as in monochorionic twins (➔ Chapter 23)
  - changes in maternal health and nutrition.
- The relevant specific resources are numerous and include:
  - metabolic substrates such as glucose, amino acids, vitamins, trace elements, oxygen
  - hormonal signals which may be stimulated by the maternal environment.
- Variation in the availability of these resources in pregnant animals can cause significant changes in the growth and development of fetal organs, sometimes with lifelong effects on their structure and function thus altering offspring phenotype.
- Epigenetic mechanisms including DNA methylation, may alter gene expression, and are therefore considered to be responsible for the altered phenotype.
- These mechanisms may allow for preferential development of essential organs, as in the 'brain-sparing effect' in growth-restricted fetuses with relatively large heads and small bodies.
- Longer-term effects of these changes are termed 'developmental programming' and may be:
  - adaptive to improve health and survival, or
  - maladaptive leading to organ dysfunction and/or disease.
- Trade-offs may also occur within organs.
- Growth-retarded fetuses may have a low nephron density compensated for by nephron hypertrophy, resulting in similarly sized kidneys to those of normal fetuses but they are more prone to early hypertension and to renal failure in later life.
- Many human diseases are thought to result from maladaptive developmental programming.
- Cardiovascular diseases which may be influenced by such programming include:
  - hypertension
  - coronary heart disease
  - stroke
  - atherosclerosis.
- Fetuses with CHD may be more vulnerable to developmental programming effects; they may have:
  - lower birth weights
  - abnormal cerebral to placental resistance ratios promoting the brain-sparing effect
  - significantly altered haemodynamics, especially in duct-dependent lesions and TGA.

Chapter 3

History and examination

History

Introduction

Assessment of the fetal cardiovascular system should begin with sufficiently accurate information to allow a detailed and full evaluation to be performed in order to permit appropriate management and counselling. Aspects of the history are considered under three headings of information that should be available before investigation is performed and in some cases before referral to a fetal cardiac clinic. Much of the following information should be available in maternity notes but specific details often need clarifying.

Parental history

Information that may influence the assessment includes:

Both parents

Relevant points to cover, using help from other relatives or interpreters if necessary:

- Clarify reason for, limitations of, and expectations from attendance.
- Consanguinity, of relevance particularly in:
    - isomeric states
    - cardiomyopathy presenting in the fetus
    - multisystem structural abnormalities.
- Presence of any of the following in either parent:
    - Autosomal dominant condition with cardiac component likely to be apparent in the fetus.
    - Autosomal dominant cardiac condition with possibility of fetal detection (e.g. long QT syndrome (LQTS)).
    - CHD—risk to fetus for CHD is variable depending on the lesion and the parent affected (➔ Chapter 2).
    - Acquired heart disease such as dilated cardiomyopathy, isolated mitral valve prolapse, and arrhythmogenic right ventricular cardiomyopathy, all of which have strong genetic components although the latter two are rarely detected in children.
- Previous child with CHD, recurrence risk dependent on cause; see ➔ Chapter 2. Ascertain diagnosis and outcome of affected case as this is important for counselling.

Maternal

Relevant points with respect to the intrauterine environment are:

- Diabetes—including present or previous gestational diabetes (➔ Chapters 19 and 24).
- Definite or suspected viral infection in 1st trimester may be relevant to structural lesions in the fetus, or later when myocarditis, cardiomyopathy, or hydrops may be consequences.
- Rubella immunity status.
- Drugs including alcohol exposure in pregnancy.
- Diseases which may impact fetal cardiovascular health:
    - Hypertension
    - Collagen vascular disease which may be subclinical and is associated with fetal heart block and myocardial dysfunction.
    - Thyrotoxicosis producing fetal tachycardia (usually sinus).

Paternal

Known factors relevant to the risk or type of CHD that are specifically father related are not clear; there is conflicting evidence on the relationship between paternal age and risk of CHD. The relationship between various types of assisted reproduction and the risk of CHD is complex; maternal or paternal factors may be important and this information is regarded as confidential thus ascertaining it as part of a clinical fetal cardiac assessment is not accepted practice.

Family history

Many pieces of information offered are not relevant to fetal risk of cardiovascular problems but often increase parental and professional awareness and anxiety. The following should be considered:

- Structural CHD in more distant than 1st-degree relative of fetus currently not thought to increase the risk, but more than one 2nd-degree relative definitely or very likely affected warrants careful thought and individual consideration.
- Acquired heart disease with genetic basis in the wider family may affect fetus, such as dilated cardiomyopathy.
- Syndromes and non-cardiac congenital abnormalities more distant than 1st-degree relative unlikely to increase risk of CHD but details should be clarified.

Rarely after careful discussion of advantages and disadvantages is it appropriate to instigate medical evaluation of other family members such as siblings of the fetus, or parental siblings. This may be sensitive and is usually better left until after the pregnancy but may be considered when the fetal diagnosis suspected is:

- LQTS (➲ p. 197)
- Complete heart block (➲ pp. 200–3)
- Marfan or more likely Loeys–Dietz syndrome as Marfan syndrome is very rarely apparent on fetal scanning, cardiac or general.

Pregnancy history

The following information should be documented if available; absence of information should also be recorded:

- Maternal hypertension, glycosuria.
- Assisted conception.
- Single or multiple; if multiple what chorionicity and amnionicity (➲ p. 244).
- Screening performed: NT, atrioventricular (AV) valve regurgitation (particularly tricuspid regurgitation (TR)) in early gestation, biochemical markers, general anomaly scan.
- Gestation and how determined.
- Any known or suspected fetal anomalies.
- Fetal karyotype.

Examination

Introduction

Parents may have medical notes and significant information is sometimes only obtained from these. It is rarely necessary to examine a parent but general observation can provide diagnostic clues relevant to fetal cardiac assessment. Parental physical signs obtained from the notes are considered on ➲ pp. 24–5 but meeting the parents in the clinic may provide additional important information.

Parental

Look out for:

- Possible syndromes previously unrecognized.
- In a fetal cardiac clinic, the following may be first suspected in a parent:
  - Noonan syndrome
  - Tuberous sclerosis
  - Alagille syndrome.
- Maternal oedema (refer to midwife/obstetrician).

Other family members

Medical physical examination of other family members will only very rarely be necessary or appropriate (➲ p. 25) and is better done by referral to a geneticist.

Chapter 4

The normal heart

Embryology

- In the first 20 days of development, the human embryo has no cardiovascular structure and nutrition is achieved by diffusion.
- Development of the heart begins in the 3rd week after fertilization and is complete by the end of week 8.
- The heart starts to beat around day 22.
- By week 12, the heart is 8mm long and has moved into the chest; thereafter it undergoes a period of growth and by 20 weeks it is 20mm long.
- The older theory of a single heart tube undergoing a series of complex folding processes has now been superseded as molecular evidence demonstrates that the primary heart tube forming in week 3 is involved in fusion with different heart fields:
  - *The first heart field* arises from the cardiac crescent and gives rise to the left ventricle.
  - *The second heart field* fuses with the primary cardiac tube and gives rise to the right ventricle and outflow tracts from its ventral portion and the atria from the dorsal portion (also referred to as the *tertiary heart field*).
- A further contribution from migrating cardiac neural crest cells enables division of the common arterial trunk into the aorta and pulmonary artery and also gives rise to the coronary circulation.
- 'Ballooning' of specific areas of the tube produces the four chambers of the heart.
- Meanwhile, looping, septation, and spiralling of the tube occur to establish a heart with normally connected vessels and with two separate sides functioning in parallel during the fetal period but able to function in series after birth.

Relevance to structural cardiac anomalies

Development of the heart is complicated and, at all stages, susceptible both to genetic and environmental factors which can modify the process and result in cardiac anomalies.

Some of these factors have been identified, e.g. those influencing the second heart field:

- Chromosome 22q11
- Maternal diabetes.

Anatomy (for echocardiography)

Introduction

A sequential approach to describing the anatomy of the heart enables a thorough echocardiographic examination to be carried out. Each chamber and vessel has its own identifying features, thus allowing recognition of each structure. Chamber and vessel identity cannot always be assumed simply by position and must, whenever possible, be defined by morphological features, many of which can be demonstrated with ultrasound.

Identification of cardiac structures enables the cardiac connections to be described. See Table 4.1 and Fig. 4.1.

Normal fetal cardiac position and axis

- The fetal heart is positioned in the left side of the chest with its apex towards the left at approximately 45 degrees to both sagittal and coronal planes.

Table 4.1 Normal cardiac connections

	Right side	Left side
Venoatrial	Superior and inferior vena cavae to right atrium	Pulmonary veins to left atrium
Atrioventricular	Right atrium to right ventricle via tricuspid valve	Left atrium to left ventricle via mitral valve
Ventricular-arterial	Right ventricle to pulmonary artery	Left ventricle to aorta

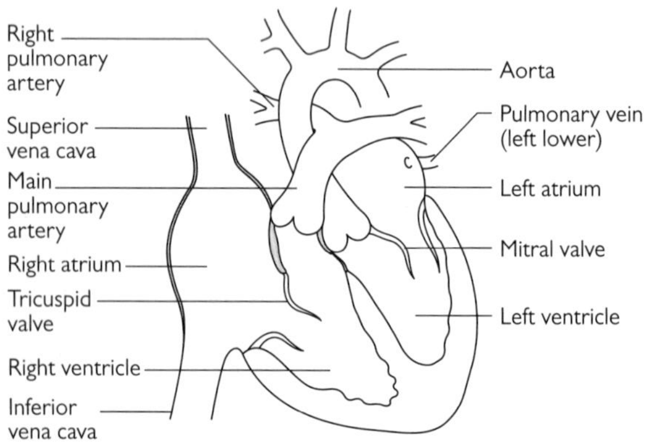

Fig. 4.1 Normal cardiac connections.

- In the normal fetus, morphologically left-sided structures lie not only to the left but also posterior to the equivalent right-sided structure.
- Thus the most posterior chamber of the heart is the left atrium, situated anterior to the spine and descending aorta.

Echocardiographic features of the cardiac chambers

Right atrium

- The venous component—a smooth-walled area into which the superior and inferior vena cavae drain, along with the coronary sinus.
- The vestibule—another smooth-walled area extending to and supporting the tricuspid valve.
- The atrial septum—comprising the floor of the oval fossa and the atrioventricular septum.
- The appendage—broad and triangular in shape, extending forward to wrap around the right wall of the aorta.
- The Eustachian valve—directing blood entering the right atrium from the inferior vena cava towards the foramen ovale.
- The coronary sinus—opening into the right atrium just above the interventricular groove.

Right ventricle

(See Table 4.2.)

- The inlet valve is the tricuspid valve which has:
  - a septal leaflet closer to the apex of the heart than the mitral valve. This produces offsetting, an important and rapid way to identify by ultrasound the tricuspid valve and right ventricle
  - tendinous cords attaching the septal leaflet to the ventricular septum.
- There is no direct continuity between the inlet valve and the arterial outlet valve.
- Has the moderator band within its cavity towards the apex.
- Shows coarser trabeculations on the septal surface than are seen in the left ventricle.
- Is anterior to the left ventricle.

Left atrium

- Is the most posterior heart chamber.
- The appendage—a tubular finger-shaped structure with a narrow opening to the left atrium.

Left ventricle

(See Table 4.2.)

- The inlet valve is a mitral valve, features of which are:
  - offsetting, being further from the apex than the tricuspid valve
  - having no tendinous attachments to the ventricular septum but only to the posterior wall via papillary muscles.
- The mitral and arterial outlet valves are in continuity through fibrous tissue.
- The ventricular septal surface has fine trabeculations.

Table 4.2 Morphological differences between right and left ventricles distinguishable on ultrasound inspection

Right ventricle	Left ventricle
Right and anterior	Left and posterior
Septal attachments of tricuspid valve	No septal attachments of mitral valve
Tricuspid valve inserted closer to apex of heart	Mitral valve inserted further from apex
Moderator band	No moderator band
Rough trabeculations	Smoother trabeculations
Tricuspid and pulmonary valves separated by muscle	Mitral and aortic valves in continuity

Echocardiographic features of the atrial and atrioventricular septa

- The atrial septum is characterized in its mid portion by the foramen ovale which:
  - provides a passage for blood from the inferior vena cava to cross to the left atrium
  - is shaped so that in normal circumstances it will flap shut after birth when left atrial pressures rise.
- The atrioventricular septum is identified by offsetting of the atrioventricular valves thereby:
  - producing an area where the left ventricle is adjacent to the right atrium
  - providing the most straightforward way to identify mitral and tricuspid valves (see Fig. 4.2).

Echocardiographic features of the ventricular septum

- The ventricular septum is mainly muscular with a small area of fibrous tissue (the perimembranous septum) in the area between the tricuspid and aortic valves.
- There are many different ways of classifying the muscular septum including:
  - inlet septum—the area between the two inlet valves and posterior to the perimembranous septum
  - apical trabecular septum—extending to the apex of the ventricles
  - outlet septum—area separating the outlet tracts of each ventricle.

Echocardiographic features of the great arteries

The key to the identification of the great arteries is their pattern of branching:

Pulmonary artery

In the fetus, the pulmonary artery divides into:

- The right pulmonary artery—a longer section is imaged than of the left, it passes under the aortic arch.

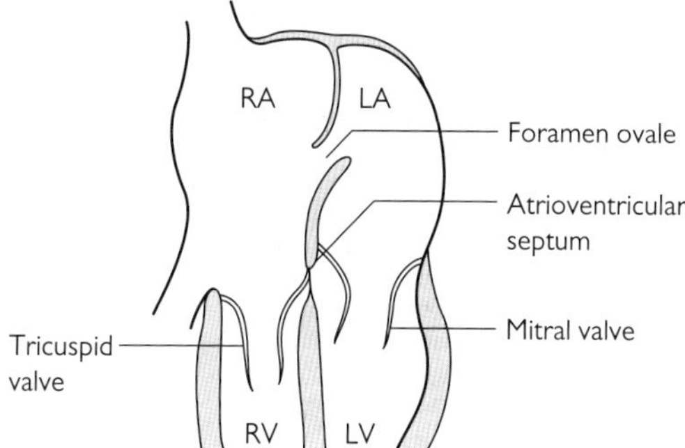

Fig. 4.2 Atrial and atrioventricular septa.

- The left pulmonary artery—a shorter section is imaged and it passes in front of the distal aortic arch.
- The arterial duct:
  - This arises from the main pulmonary artery at the point of branching.
  - It is larger than the branch pulmonary arteries.
  - It connects the pulmonary artery directly to the descending aorta distal to the origin of the left subclavian artery (for aberrant origin of aortic arch vessels, especially of the right subclavian artery, see ➲ Chapter 6).

Aorta

The aorta comprises the ascending aorta, the arch (curving to the left of the trachea), and the descending aorta. See ➲ pp. 101–2 for right aortic arch.

- Its origin (and valve) lie behind, to the right and at right angles to the pulmonary valve in a normally connected heart.
- The ascending aorta gives rise to the left and right coronary arteries just above the aortic valve.
- The transverse arch gives rise to three main branches:
  - The right brachiocephalic artery giving rise to the right subclavian and right common carotid arteries.
  - The left common carotid.
  - The left subclavian artery.
- Aortic branches are significantly further from the aortic valve than the pulmonary artery trifurcation is from the pulmonary valve.
- The aortic isthmus extends from the left subclavian artery to where the ductus arteriosus inserts into the descending aorta. It is the narrowest part of the aortic arch.
- The descending aorta is to the left of the spine and posterior to the inferior vena cava at the level of the diaphragm.

The fetal circulation

Introduction

- The concentration of haemoglobin is greater in the fetus than in the postnatal circulation (by 50%).
- In addition, fetal haemoglobin has a greater affinity for oxygen compared to adult haemoglobin.
- These differences permit fetal well-being with left ventricular and ascending aortic blood oxygen saturation in the region of 60%.
- In the fetus, oxygenation of blood takes place in the placenta.
- The fetal circulation preferentially supplies vital organs with highly oxygenated blood returning from the placenta while allowing only a small amount of blood to reach the lungs.

The circulation

The haemodynamic objectives in the fetus are achieved by three pathways (see Fig. 4.3 and Table 4.3) which close after birth.

The venous duct

- Half of the well-oxygenated umbilical venous blood avoids the liver and enters the inferior vena cava via the venous duct.
- This blood streams preferentially through the foramen ovale to the left atrium as a result of:
  - direction and speed of blood flow in the venous duct
  - angle of flow into the right atrium created by the Eustachian valve.

The foramen ovale

- In the normal heart, the foramen ovale is usually kept open by the mechanisms previously described and by the lower pressure found in the left atrium compared to the right atrium.
- In disease states, patency may be reduced with important consequences.

The arterial duct

- High vascular resistance in unaerated lungs directs up to 80% of blood in the main pulmonary artery into the arterial duct and then into the descending aorta and lower body.
- The remaining 20% passes via the pulmonary artery branches to the lungs and then returns to the left atrium via four pulmonary veins.
- Coronary arteries and head and neck vessels arise from the aorta before ductal blood enters and thus are supplied with the most oxygen-rich arterial blood.
- The descending aorta is post ductal and therefore the least well-oxygenated arterial blood serves the lower body and returns blood to the placenta via two umbilical arteries.
- At around 28–32 weeks, flow to the lungs increases while that in the ductus venosus and through the foramen ovale is reduced in preparation for postnatal changes.

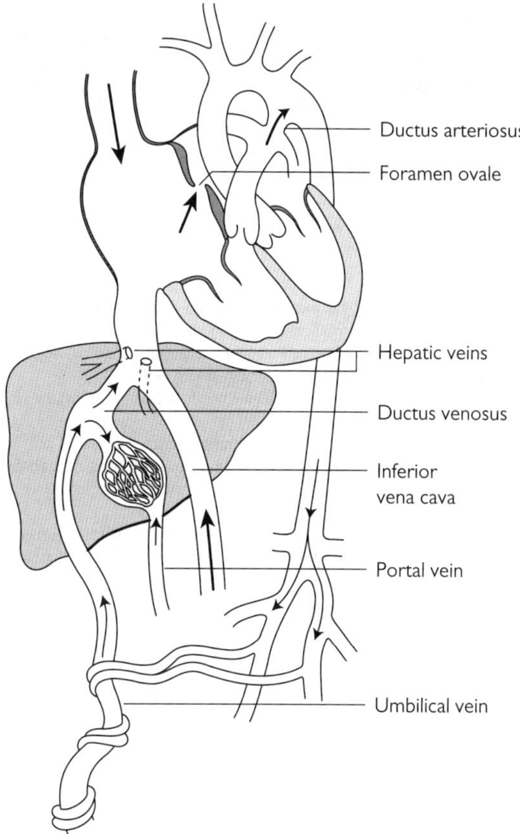

Fig. 4.3 Normal fetal circulation showing fetal pathways as discussed in the text. (Note: the anatomical relationship shown between the ductus venosus, portal vein, and hepatic vein is only approximate.)

Table 4.3 Summary of fetal pathways

Fetal pathway	Anatomical position	Haemodynamic objective
Ductus venosus	Umbilical vein to inferior vena cava	To bypass liver
Foramen ovale	Right atrium to left atrium	To fill left heart
Ductus arteriosus	Main pulmonary artery to aorta	To bypass lungs

Physiological variations

The normal fetal circulation has previously been described. The presence of two parallel circulations (pulmonary and systemic) with pathways for shunting between them allows changes in organ blood flow during gestation in response to various stimuli, both normal and pathological. Where necessary, these aspects are discussed in the text.

The ability of the fetal heart to function effectively as a pump depends on intrinsic factors (myocardial performance) and extrinsic ones such as preload and afterload. These factors are considered in more detail in the sections on assessing function (➔ Chapter 18) and on hydrops (➔ Chapter 22).

Changes at birth

- At birth, the function of gas exchange is taken over by the lungs.
- Conversion from fetal (umbilical-placental) circulation to postnatal (pulmonary) circulation involves important changes including closure of the fetal shunts that are no longer required (Fig. 4.4).
- When the lungs aerate, there is a 10-fold reduction in pulmonary vascular resistance, thus:
  - pulmonary blood flow increases, causing left atrial pressure to rise
  - right-to-left shunting through the foramen ovale ceases or transiently reverses (right atrial pressure falls as the venous duct closes)
  - systemic arterial oxygen saturation rises
  - closure of the ductus arteriosus commences, taking up to 4 days to close and sometimes longer, especially in significantly preterm infants with respiratory disease.

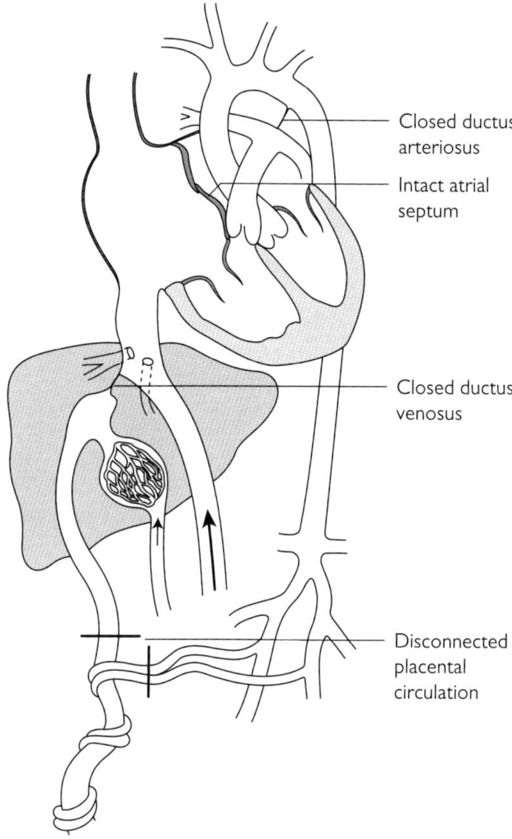

Fig. 4.4 Postnatal circulation after closure of fetal pathways.

Chapter 5

Indications for fetal echocardiography

Introduction

- The incidence of structural CHD is 8:1000 live births:
  - For counselling purposes, the figure of approximately 1% is used.
- The incidence is higher in the prenatal population, with cardiac diagnoses biased towards:
  - more complicated lesions
  - those also having rhythm disturbances
  - those with associated non-cardiac anomalies including structural and chromosomal abnormalities.
- The general anomaly scan screens for CHD in a low-risk population.
- 'Suspected abnormal' as an indication for detailed echocardiography produces the highest yield for abnormalities.

Indications for a detailed cardiac scan

Factors known to increase the risk for heart disease are indications to offer a detailed cardiac scan and are summarized in Table 5.1.

Table 5.1 Indications for a fetal cardiac scan

Indication	Risk to fetus for CHD
Structural abnormality suspected at the anomaly scan	High
Previous child (or fetus) with CHD	2–3% 10% if 2 previously affected
Parent with CHD:	
maternal	6% (higher for left-sided lesions)
paternal	2–3%
Maternal diabetes:	
type 1	3–5%
type 2	Less well defined, depends on HbA1c in 1st trimester
gestational	Probably not increased
Increased nuchal translucency	5–10% (➲ Chapter 21) Increases with increased measurement
Abnormal cardiac axis	High
Other structural anomaly with cardiac associations (Table 5.2)	Variable
At risk of syndrome with cardiac associations (➲ Chapter 2)	Variable
Monochorionic twins (mono- and diamniotic)	4–11% (for at least 1 of set) for MCDA, higher for MCMA
Exposure to teratogen: some anticonvulsants alcohol lithium retinoic acid	Variable
Hydrops (and isolated pleural + pericardial effusions)	Variable
Abnormal cardiac rhythm Fast/slow/persistently irregular	Variable
Maternal anti-Ro/anti-La antibodies	2–3% for complete heart block Small risk of myocarditis
Use of maternal NSAIDs	Variable, gestation dependent (ductal constriction)

Table 5.1 (*Contd*)

Indication	Risk to fetus for CHD
Abnormal fetal karyotype (➲ Chapter 2)	Variable but high
Maternal phenylketonuria	Up to 8–10% Depending on control
Parent with autosomal dominant cardiac condition	Most not detectable in the fetus
Some maternal infections (including parvovirus)	Evidence of myocarditis or fetal anaemia
Absence of the ductus venosus	High association with cardiac anomalies—structural and functional
Hyperdynamic situations including: arteriovenous anomalies vascular tumours	May develop heart failure

Note

- A 1st-degree relative of the fetus is:
  - A parent, or
  - A sibling
- Relatives of the fetus more distant than 1st-degree with CHD are not considered to increase the risk to the fetus.
- Some cardiomyopathies have an unclear familial pattern and more distant relatives may be relevant:
  - Fetal diagnosis is uncommon and a normal study does not exclude the diagnosis.
  - In many cases fetal cardiac assessment is not indicated.
  - Discussion with the parent's cardiologist may help guide pre- and postnatal management.
- Using fetal echocardiography to avoid invasive testing is unreliable:
  - Only 50% of fetuses with Down syndrome will have a detectable cardiac lesion.
- The highest yield for structural CHD is in the apparently 'low-risk' population where an abnormality is suspected:
  - Thus the importance of screening.

Non-cardiac structural anomalies associated with increased risk of CHD

- Some non-cardiac structural lesions are associated with increased risk for CHD (see Table 5.2):
  - Even if the karyotype is normal.
  - Some will have syndromic associations.
- Microarray and other genetic advances now provide more information; this is discussed in detail in ➲ Chapters 2 and 8.

Table 5.2 Non-cardiac anomalies and commonly associated cardiac lesions

Congenital diaphragmatic hernia	VSD Tetralogy of Fallot
Exomphalos	VSD Tetralogy of Fallot
Duodenal atresia —and other bowel atresias	VSD AVSD
Tracheo-oesophageal fistula	VSD Tetralogy of Fallot
Cystic hygroma	Left-sided obstructive lesions
Some upper limb anomalies	Variable
Hydrops	Structure, function or rhythm

Chapter 6

Fetal echocardiography

Introduction

- In spite of improvements in technology and education, around 50% of CHD remains undetected in the fetus.
- Improved postnatal outcome following fetal detection has now been demonstrated for many cardiac lesions, emphasizing the value of prenatal diagnosis.
- A systematic approach to screening and detailed assessment is essential so that every structure is examined regardless of fetal position or mobility.
- Traditionally the 4-chamber view has been the basis of the fetal cardiac examination.
- The 3-vessel trachea view (see ➔ Chapter 7) is now also standard for screening at the anomaly scan.
- A logical sequential approach for identifying normal cardiac connections, as described in ➔ Chapter 4, can be used.
- This chapter addresses the requirements for the screening examination of the low-risk population and also fetal echocardiography for those considered to be at an increased risk as well as those in whom an abnormality is suspected.

Clinical application of relevant physics

- The physics of ultrasound is covered in detail in many textbooks, including the *Oxford Specialist Handbook in Echocardiography*.
- This brief overview serves to highlight principles with practical relevance to obtaining optimal fetal cardiac images and Doppler information.

Greyscale 2D image

This is the basis for all examinations; image quality may be improved by applying the following techniques:

- Choice of probe is important and varies according to the distance of the fetus from the probe, as influenced by various factors.
- High-frequency probes, e.g. 6–8 MHz, provide higher resolution and thus clearer images but have less penetration; they are therefore good for early pregnancy and normal pregnancies but may be less helpful for later gestations, obese mothers, or in the presence of polyhydramnios:
    - In these situations, a 3–4 MHz probe may be more useful.
- Better images are obtained if the angle of insonation is as near as possible to a right angle to the structure under scrutiny, in contrast to Doppler assessment (see below).
- Image resolution may be improved by:
    - reducing the sector size of image zone
    - adjusting the focal zone to the level of interrogation
    - applying the zoom so that the heart image occupies at least half of the screen
    - use of harmonics.
- Cineloop facilities are helpful to review images slowly in all phases of the cardiac cycle.
- Safety should be considered but most ultrasound machines have mechanisms which prevent safe limits being exceeded.

Doppler

- The following Doppler modalities are available on most ultrasound machines:
    - Pulsed wave (PW) Doppler
    - Colour Doppler
    - Continuous wave (CW) Doppler.
- The principle behind Doppler is that the frequency of ultrasound changes when it is scattered by a moving target—the Doppler shift.
- This change is related to the speed of movement of the target.
- If the frequency of the emitted beam is known and that of the beam received is detected then the Doppler shift can be displayed as the velocity of the moving target (either blood cells or heart structure).

Pulsed wave Doppler

- See Fig. 6.1.
- Allows for accurate measurement of speed and direction of blood flow.
- The angle of insonation should be small, as near to parallel to the direction of blood flow as possible.
- The sample volume can be placed in a specific position so that the velocity at that particular point in the heart can be measured accurately.
- Its main disadvantage is that it can only sample velocities up to a certain speed and thus is not useful if velocities are high.

Colour Doppler

- See Fig. 6.2.
- Is another way of displaying PW information.

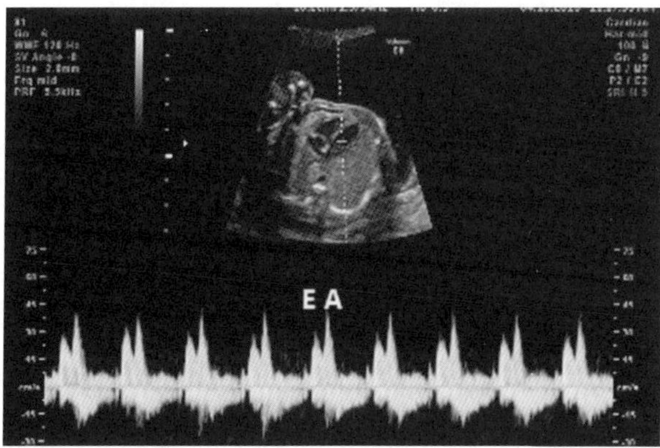

Fig. 6.1 PW signal from LV inlet taken from 4-chamber view. Note Doppler cursor in line with direction of blood flow (small angle of insonation), forward flow to LV shows normal E (early) and A (late, atrial contraction) configuration and velocities.

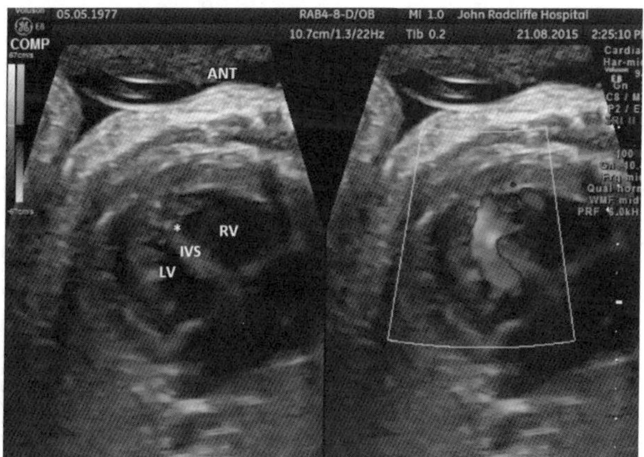

Fig. 6.2 Colour flow Doppler interrogation of interventricular septum (IVS) in 4-chamber view making presence of 1 or more VSDs much clearer than image alone. In colour, signal was blue indicating flow from right (RV) to left ventricle (LV). (See colour plate section).

- Is useful for adding to information obtained from 2D imaging to demonstrate:
  - direction of blood flow
  - speed of flow
  - patency of valves
  - regurgitation through valves
  - abnormal flow, e.g. across the ventricular septum.
- Power Doppler signal reflects wave amplitude not velocity and is thus less influenced by angle of insonation.
- When power Doppler is combined with high-density colour Doppler, the displayed signal incorporates direction of flow and is good for demonstrating low-velocity flow in small vessels.

Continuous wave Doppler

- See Fig. 6.3.
- CW Doppler can accurately measure and quantify high velocities.
- It continuously emits and receives information from all moving targets and, unlike PW Doppler, cannot determine exactly where the accelerated jet arises and so this needs to be established first, by using a combination of 2D imaging, colour Doppler, and PW Doppler.

M-mode

- See Fig. 6.4.
- Is useful in the assessment of fetal arrhythmias by giving a visual demonstration of the relationship between atrial and ventricular contraction.
- It can also be used to measure ventricular and myocardial dimensions and function.

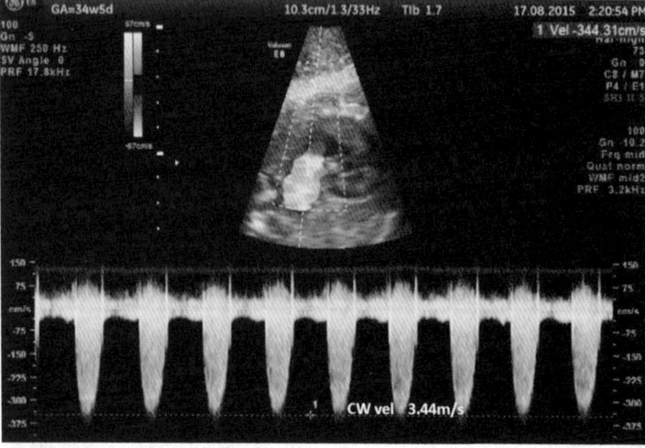

Fig. 6.3 Outlet view of LV with colour flow Doppler highlighting high velocity in right ventricular outflow tract (LVOT). CW confirms velocity of 3.44 m/sec with good angle of insonation indicating severe AS (peak instantaneous gradient from modified Bernoulli equation 47 mmHg).

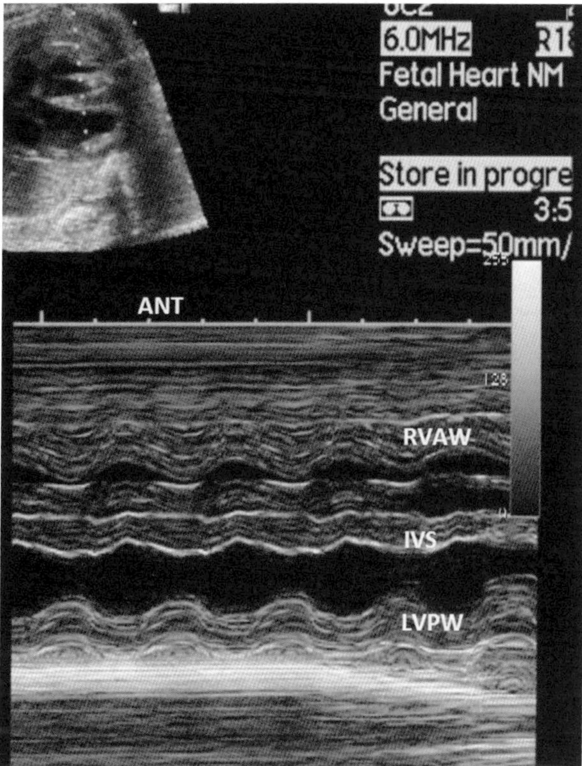

Fig. 6.4 Enlarged M-mode examination obtained with cursor at right angles to right ventricular anterior wall (RVAW), interventricular septum (IVS), and left ventricular posterior wall (LVPW) as seen on the 2D inset image. Measurements of muscle thickness and cavity size can be made on the M-mode trace. Calculations of systolic function can be performed if relevant.

General principles of cardiac scanning

Certain points are important to every scan performed.

Communication

Before the scan, there should be an explanation to the parents about:
- why the scan is being performed
- the limitations of antenatal cardiac assessment.

It is helpful to be aware of parental expectations and understanding.

Image quality

Factors which influence image quality include:
- gestation
- fetal position
- maternal size
- poly/oligohydramnios
- multiple pregnancy
- quality of equipment and familiarity of operator with equipment.

The normal fetal circulation

- The following anatomical features influence interpretation of the fetal scan:
    - foramen ovale
    - ductus arteriosus
    - ductus venosus
- All are part of the normal fetal circulation and programmed to close postnatally:
    - Their closure cannot be predicted antenatally.
- Some abnormalities, e.g. coarctation of the aorta, may only present postnatally when the shunts close and therefore cannot be excluded antenatally.
- Some lesions evolve during pregnancy and become more obvious in later pregnancy.

Screening examination of the heart

The UK Fetal Anomaly Screening Programme (FASP) applies to the examination of all aspects of the fetus and is regularly updated. From the cardiac perspective, there has been much time committed to improving screening with the aim of increasing the antenatal detection of CHD. The International Society of Ultrasound in Obstetrics and Gynecology has also published guidelines on this subject.

- It is essential that nothing is assumed in the examination of the fetal heart.
- Everything must be proved, including left and right sides of the fetus.
- Every chamber and every vessel have their own identifying features.
- Following a protocol, demonstration of substantially normal cardiac anatomy can usually be achieved.

The cardiac protocol in FASP guidelines published in June 2015 includes the following views at 18–22 weeks:

1. Situs/laterality

- Heart and stomach should be on the left side of the fetus.
- At the level of the diaphragm:
  - The aorta should be on the left
  - The IVC is anterior to it and to the right of the spine (Fig. 6.5)

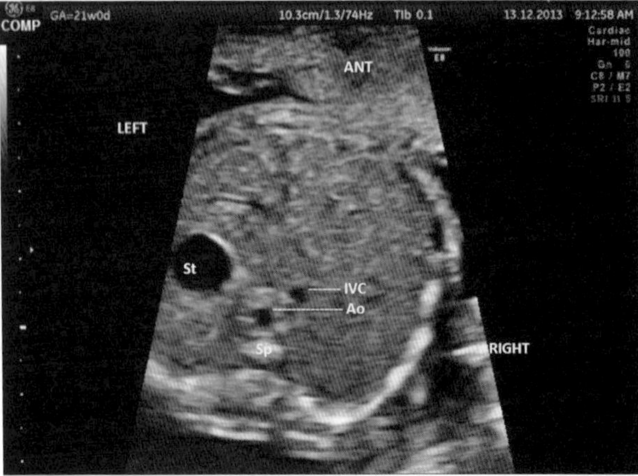

Fig. 6.5 Cross-sectional image at level of diaphragm allowing situs solitus to be identified providing fetal orientation is as indicated.

2. Four-chamber view

This should be as a transverse section through the thorax to include a complete rib (Fig. 6.6) and show the following:

- The heart is mostly in the left chest.
- The apex is to the left at an angle of 30–60 degrees to the sagittal axis.
- The heart occupies ⅓ of the chest, subjective assessment is usually sufficient but area (A) can be measured if there is doubt and should be no more than ⅓ or circumference (C) no more than ½ of chest measurement in ventricular diastole (➔ Fig. 18.2, p. 209).
- This measurement may include a physiological pericardial effusion, less than 3 mm in maximum depth at any point and in any phase of the cardiac cycle.
- 2 atria are equal in size.
- 2 ventricles are equal in size.
- 2 AV valves open freely with each cycle.
- The 2 AV valves should meet at the crux as an offset cross:
    - The valve closest to the apex is the tricuspid valve.
    - The valve furthest from the apex is the mitral valve.
    - The valves define the ventricles, thus TV will identify the RV, MV the LV.
- The RV morphology includes a moderator band (MB) near the apex.
- The ventricular septum is intact.
- The foramen ovale opens into the left atrium.
- The rhythm is regular at a rate of 120–160 bpm.

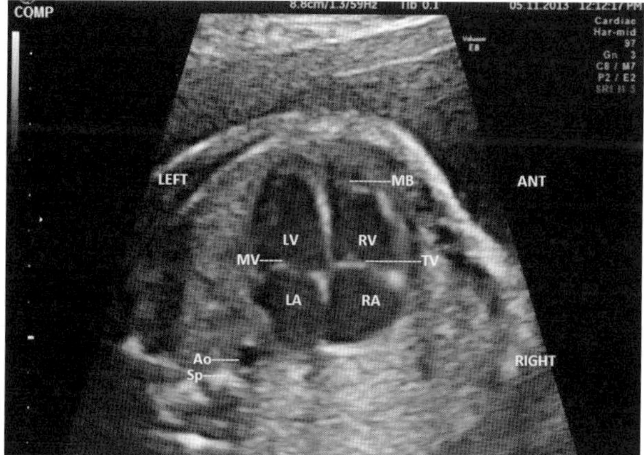

Fig. 6.6 Normal 4-chamber view.

3. Aorta/left ventricular outflow tract

- See Fig. 6.7.
- The aorta can be identified as it gives rise to head and neck vessels.
- Sweeps out towards the right shoulder.
- And then turns through 90 degrees to pass to the left side of the trachea.
- The anterior wall of the aorta is continuous with the ventricular septum.

4. Pulmonary/right ventricular outflow tract

- See Figs 6.8a and 6.8b.
- The pulmonary artery (PA) is identified by its division into 3 branches:
  - left pulmonary artery (LPA)
  - right pulmonary artery (RPA)
  - ductus arteriosus (DA).
- It passes straight backwards towards the spine.
- The PA should be slightly bigger than the aorta.
- The main PA continues as the ductus arteriosus to join the aorta.
- The great arteries should cross over each other.

5. Three-vessel trachea (3VT) view

- A transverse view of the upper mediastinum to demonstrate the main PA continuing as the ductus to join the transverse aortic arch on the left side of the trachea, SVC to the right (see ➲ Chapter 7).

At present the use of colour Doppler is not part of the screening examination but saving images, preferably moving images, is now standard practice.

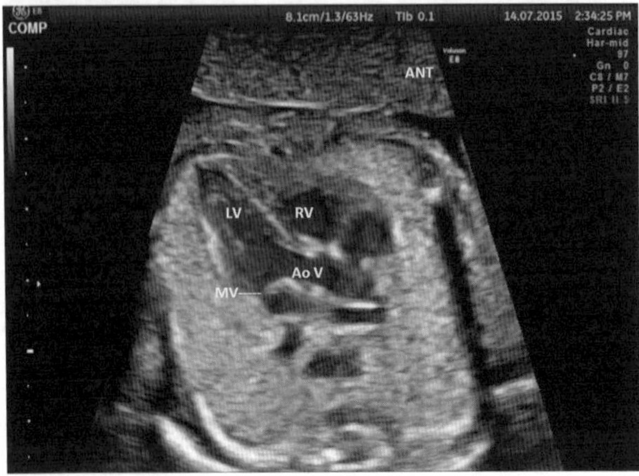

Fig. 6.7 Long-axis view of LVOT in systole showing continuity between IVS through the aortic valve (AoV) to ascending aorta.

(a)

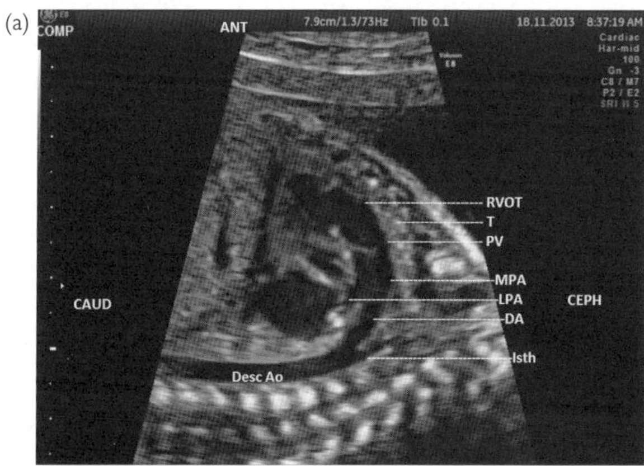

(b)

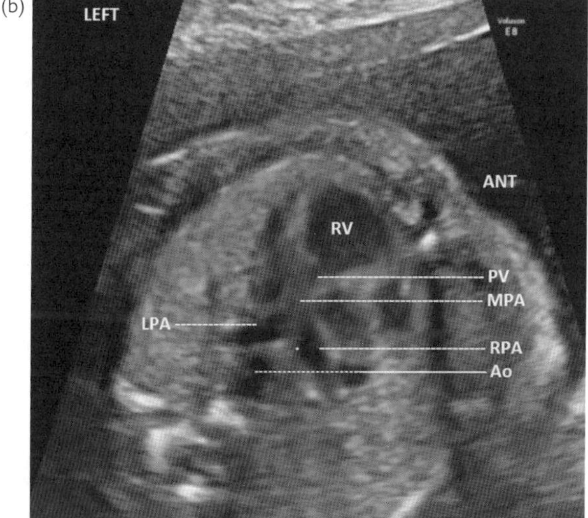

Fig. 6.8 (a) Oblique cut through right ventricular outflow tract (RVOT) showing PV, PA, LPA, DA, and aortic isthmus (Isth). (b) Cephalad angulation from 4-chamber view showing PA with confluent RPA and LPA.

Helpful observations

- The most posterior chamber of the heart is the left atrium.
- The descending aorta lies between spine and left atrium.
- The right ventricle is bigger than left, especially in 3rd trimester.
- IVC and SVC should be seen draining into the RA.
- A normal 4-chamber view will exclude most uncorrectable cardiac lesions and up to ⅓ of significant cardiac anomalies (Box 6.1).
- Outlet views increase the range of abnormalities detected (Box 6.2).
- By the end of the examination, 'normal cardiac connections' should have been defined see ➲ Chapter 4.

Alternative approach to screening assessment

- 5 transverse views are obtained having established laterality.
- 5 views are obtained as follows:
  - V1: transverse view of the fetal abdomen to demonstrate situs.
  - V2: 4-chamber view of heart.
  - V3: 5-chamber view demonstrating aortic root arising from left ventricle (extended 4-chamber view).
  - V4: to demonstrate bifurcation of pulmonary artery.
  - V5: 3VT view with trachea at level of main PA joining the ductus arteriosus.

Box 6.1 Cardiac lesions resulting in an abnormal 4-chamber view

- Ebstein's anomaly/dysplastic tricuspid valve
- Tricuspid/mitral atresia
- AVSD—complete and partial
- Hypoplastic left heart syndrome
- Pulmonary atresia with intact septum
- Double inlet left ventricle
- Congenitally corrected transposition
- Large ventricular septal defect (inlet/muscular)
- Cardiac tumours
- Laterality defects
- Severe aortic/pulmonary stenosis or atresia.

Box 6.2 Cardiac lesions detected using great artery views

- Tetralogy of Fallot
- Pulmonary atresia with VSD
- DORV
- Transposition of great arteries
- Common arterial trunk
- Some cases of coarctation
- Pulmonary/aortic stenosis.

Detailed fetal echocardiography

- The aim of fetal echocardiography is to provide a complete assessment of anatomy and function in pregnancies at increased risk of or thought to have a cardiac abnormality on screening.
- This examination involves of all of the earlier described techniques in this chapter.
- In addition, fetal echocardiography involves the use of all Doppler modalities in order to further assess:
    - situs and cardiac axis
    - all 4 cardiac chambers, septa, and both great vessels
    - systemic and pulmonary venous return
    - cardiac rhythm and function.

Functional assessment

A detailed scan should include colour Doppler assessment of valves, the DA, and the ventricular septum. Any abnormal velocity, direction of flow, or turbulence warrants detailed PW Doppler evaluation. Rhythm, muscle function, and detailed measurements may be indicated.

Normal values

Detailed dimensions are sometimes important; these are related to gestation and can be quantified using Z-scores.

Limitations

- Not all cardiac anomalies are detectable antenatally; this needs to be shared with the parents.
- Fetal shunts are normal.
- Some valvar anomalies may not be present early in pregnancy and evolve such that they may only become apparent in late pregnancy or postnatally:
  - Mild AS
  - Mild PS
  - Even tetralogy of Fallot.
- Some lesions can only be diagnosed with confidence or excluded postnatally when the shunts close.

Advanced ultrasound imaging

- Spatiotemporal image correlation (STIC) which uses automated transverse and longitudinal sweeps of the anterior chest wall is the current method used to acquire 3D/4D images of the fetal heart.
- The 3D automated volume acquisition consists of multiple 2D slices which are combined to create one complete moving 3D cardiac cycle, which is called a 4D volume data set, in which the 4th dimension is time.
- Each of these virtual planes can be moved, rotated, and analysed.
- STIC has been used in conjunction with inversion mode and B-flow imaging.
- Inversion mode in which the 3D pixels (voxels) of the greyscale images are inverted has been used in an attempt to make structures more discernible.
- B-flow imaging is used to improve the weak signals reflected from the blood and suppresses strong signals from surrounding structures:
    - This has been used to improve the identification of small-calibre, low-velocity vessels such as pulmonary veins.
- Drop-out artefact and reverberations occur frequently. The image will be affected by the same elements which create suboptimal 2D imaging, such as oligohydramnios and maternal obesity.
- The image may also be affected by fetal breathing or fetal movement during acquisition.

Applications

Diagnostic

Suggested benefits of 3D imaging include the following:

- Identification of papillary muscle and attachments.
- Delineation of VSDs.
- Identification of semi-lunar valve morphology:
    - Including when fetal intervention is being considered.
- Identification of the atrial appendages in suspected atrial isomerism.
- Assessment of cardiac function:
    - Reference values for ventricular volumes and ejection fraction have been developed using virtual organ computer-aided analysis (VOCAL) and have been used in the management of fetuses with growth restriction and twin-to-twin transfusion.

Whether or not advanced imaging improves antenatal diagnosis is still unclear:

- It is time-consuming.
- There are not enough studies to support or refute the benefit of this imaging modality.
- It has been suggested that 3D/4D imaging may benefit telemedicine and off-line analysis.
- A STIC image may be acquired by an examiner at a remote site and be reviewed offline, this may be useful in areas with limited access to detailed fetal echocardiography.

Training and support

Training of sonographers in fetal cardiac examination using STIC may allow them to improve their understanding of the fetal heart, specifically the spatial relationship of heart structures.

Chapter 7

Three-vessel trachea view

Introduction

The three vessel trachea (3VT) view has recently been introduced as one of the views required as part of the screening examination of the heart at the routine anomaly scan (➔ Chapter 6).

The aim of this view is to increase detection of duct-dependent cardiac lesions, thereby optimizing neonatal management of babies born with CHD.

The normal three-vessel trachea view

- This view can be achieved even in the 1st trimester.
- It is achieved by obtaining a 4-chamber view and then scanning anteriorly to show the LVOT followed by RVOT and continuing this sweep to obtain the 3VT section.
- It is thus a transverse view of the upper mediastinum a few millimetres cephalad to the formerly used 3-vessel screening view showing:
  - transverse main PA
  - transverse aortic arch and isthmus
  - cross-section of the trachea (a white circular structure with a black lumen)
  - cross section of the SVC
  - the connection of the DA to the aortic arch.
- The initial assessment should use 2D imaging.
- This can be followed by the use of colour Doppler to add important information about direction of flow.
- A normal 3VT view shows:
  - PA diameter slightly bigger than the aorta
  - aorta diameter slightly bigger than SVC
  - PA and DA pass to the left of the trachea
  - aorta also passes to the left of the trachea to meet the DA as a 'V'
  - colour Doppler shows flow is anteroposterior in the Ao, PA, and DA
  - no arterial vessel is seen to the right of the trachea
  - there should be a space between the anterior border of the vessels and the back of the sternum, occupied by the thymus.
- The thymus is:
  - slightly less echogenic than the lungs
  - bordered either side by the mammary arteries.
- Various methods are used to assess the size of the thymus including
  - thymic:thoracic ratio (T:T ratio)
  - area
  - circumference.
- The T:T ratio is obtained by dividing the distance from the anterior of the transverse aorta to the posterior of the sternum (i.e. the diameter of thymus) by the intrathoracic diameter (see Fig. 7.1).
- T:T ratio can be related to gestational age although some consider it to be constant throughout pregnancy with a value of 0.44.
- T:T measurement of <0.3, indicative of a small thymus, is particularly associated with 22q11 deletion, especially in the presence of a conotruncal anomaly.
- A small thymus may also be seen with
  - Trisomy 18 and 21
  - intrauterine growth restriction
  - chorioamnionitis.

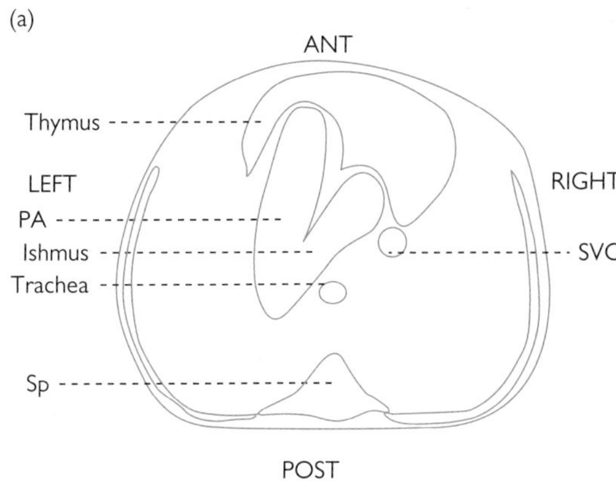

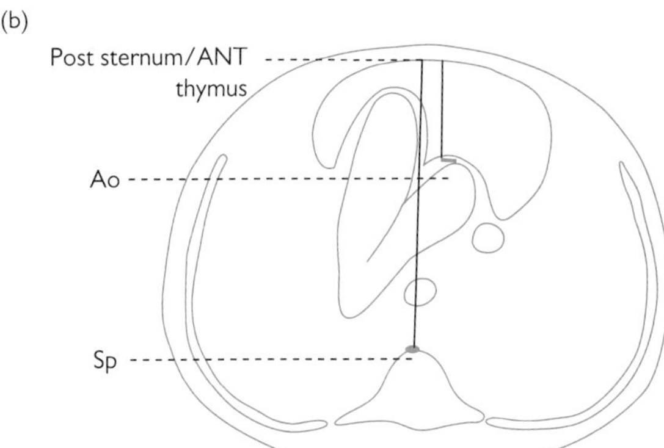

Fig. 7.1 (a) Diagram of 3VT view. (b) Diagram of 3VT view showing measurements for TT ratio. In practice, the front of thymus and back of sternum are usually hard to distinguish.

Abnormalities of the 3VT view

The 3VT view can be abnormal because of an abnormality in:

- Vessel number
- Vessel size
- Vessel relationship to trachea
- Direction of flow.

These arrangements are summarized in ➔ Table 15.4, p. 170.

Lesions likely to produce an abnormal 3VT view

Left-sided lesions

- HLHS
- Severe AS
- Aortic atresia
- Coarctation of the aorta
- Interrupted aortic arch.

Right-sided lesions

- Pulmonary atresia
- PS
- Tetralogy of Fallot
- Ebstein's
- Dysplastic TV
- Tricuspid atresia.

Mixed

- TGA
- Common arterial trunk.

Chapter 8

Other investigations

Introduction

It is important to determine whether a cardiac lesion is:

- isolated, or
- associated with non-cardiac abnormalities, or
- part of a syndrome (➔ Chapter 2).

This information is important:

- to allow accurate counselling about fetal prognosis for both cardiac and non-cardiac diagnoses
- for management of pregnancy and delivery
- in determining recurrence risk and management of subsequent pregnancies
- in case assessment of parents and other family members should be offered
- some genetic information can only be obtained by invasive testing
- the method of obtaining material for genetic testing and the method of analysis depends on gestation, the level of risk (of both the procedure and of an abnormal result) as well as on patient choice.

Invasive testing

All invasive tests are associated with a small increased chance of miscarriage and include the following:

- Amniocentesis
- Chorionic villus sampling (CVS)
- Fetal blood sampling.

These tests provide samples for testing:

- Chromosome number and structure
- Single gene disorders
- Biochemistry (e.g. for metabolic disease such as Smith–Lemli–Opitz syndrome, associated with AVSD).

Amniocentesis

- Can be performed from about 15 weeks' gestation and at any stage later in pregnancy.
- Involves taking 10–20 mL of amniotic fluid transabdominally under ultrasound guidance.
- Fetal cells in the amniotic fluid are grown in culture and prepared for chromosome analysis.
- Molecular genetic testing can also be performed to test for the chromosomes (microarray, FISH, quantitative fluorescence polymerase chain reaction).
- DNA can be extracted from the cultured sample to test for single gene disorders.
- The miscarriage risk associated with the procedure is about 0.5%.

Chorionic villus sampling

- Can be performed from 11 weeks' gestation.
- A small sample of placenta from the villous area of the chorion is obtained by transabdominal or transcervical access under ultrasound guidance.
- Karyotyping, direct molecular testing, or DNA extraction can be performed following culture of the sample.
- The available tests are the same as for amniocentesis.
- There is a small possibility of confined placental mosaicism giving false results.
- The miscarriage risk associated with the procedure is about 0.5–1%.

Fetal blood sampling

- The sample is usually obtained from the umbilical cord at the point of placental insertion.
- This higher-risk procedure is almost exclusively performed if blood is needed for other investigations such as fetal anaemia or during fetocide to store DNA for future analysis.

Genetic testing of invasive samples

These samples can be used for testing for chromosomal or single gene disorders.

Chromosome tests

Microarray testing

- Comparative genome hybridization is generally used.
- This allows specific probes to attach to the chromosomes to detect whether there are regions deleted or duplicated.
- Resolution depends on the number of probes, e.g. 60,000 probes give about a 60 kb resolution.
- Takes about 14 days.
- Can be performed more quickly on DNA extracted directly from a CVS sample.
- The advantage is that it is twice as good as conventional karyotyping in detecting chromosomal disorders.
- The disadvantage is that incidental findings and variants of unknown significance can be identified which may complicate the explanation to the parents.

Karyotype

- Takes about 10–14 days to obtain results as cells have to be cultured to obtain metaphase, the appropriate stage in cell division to examine the chromosomes under the microscope.
- The resolution is 5–10 Mb.
- Although microarray is now the method of choice, karyotyping is used to identify translocations and chromosomal rearrangements and may help to clarify the microarray results.

Fluorescence in situ hybridization (FISH)

- A small number of specific probes enable deletions or duplications to be identified.
- Only a small number of probes are usually used in one test.
- The technique has now largely been replaced by microarrays.
- May be useful if a specific rapid answer is required.
- Also used when performing follow-up parental chromosome testing when a chromosome variant is identified in the fetus.

Quantitative fluorescence polymerase chain reaction (QF-PCR)

- Is a more rapid test and can be performed in 1–2 days.
- Involves using a DNA marker to map a specific area of chromosome using probes.
- Generally used to detect aneuploidies, including of the sex chromosomes and triploidy.
- Can be used to detect specific single gene mutations, e.g. for Noonan syndrome but is rarely used in practice.
- This test is currently offered to women with a higher-risk result (>1:150) following Down syndrome screening.
    - Soon to be replaced by maternal cell-free fetal DNA testing (cffDNA, ➔ p. 74)

Molecular genetic testing

- These tests can be performed for single gene disorders and use the DNA extracted from cultured amniocentesis or CVS samples.
- Testing can also be performed directly on DNA extracted from CVS samples.

Conventional Sanger sequencing

- This test sequences the DNA code of each gene.
- It can be used to test for particular familial mutations in pregnancy.
- It can also be used to investigate the cause of malformations in a fetus, but this may be impractical during pregnancy as it can take weeks to complete.
- Is also used to test parental blood samples to determine recurrence risks.

Gene panel tests

- Next-generation sequencing techniques allow more than one gene to be tested at once.
- These gene panels are becoming more available.
- May be used in future to investigate anomalies where the cause is known to be heterogeneous such as:
  - Noonan syndrome
  - cardiomyopathy
  - heterotaxy
- Can also be performed following a pregnancy to help determine the diagnosis and recurrence risks.

Whole exome and whole genome sequencing

- Next-generation sequencing techniques allow the genes to be sequenced at once (whole exome sequencing) or the entire genome to be sequenced in one test (whole genome sequencing).
- This allows diagnoses to be made which have not first been clinically suspected.
- Is likely to become more available in future to identify the cause of many fetal anomalies.
- Results may make counselling more complex.

Non-invasive genetic testing

- Involves testing the small amount of fetal DNA present in the maternal circulation.
- This cell-free fetal DNA (cffDNA) originates from the placenta.
- The amount of fetal DNA increases with increases in gestation.
- Testing can be performed from about 9–10 weeks' gestation.
- The advantage of cffDNA testing is that the miscarriage risk associated with invasive testing is avoided.
- It allows examination for certain aneuploidies, currently trisomy 21, trisomy 13, and trisomy 18.
- These are considered to be screening tests.
- There is a low false-positive rate (due to confined placental mosaicism) and false-negative rate.
- Invasive testing is offered to confirm a positive result.
- Other chromosomal deletions and duplications (e.g. 22q11 deletion and XO) can be tested by this method but are less accurate and currently not widely used.
- Single gene disorders can be tested for using this method, e.g. Noonan syndrome. This may be offered in some circumstances as a bespoke test where a specific mutation is known in a family.
- Other single gene disorder tests are available as an cffDNA panel test and these will become more widely available:
  - No confirmatory invasive test is required as the accuracy is high.
- Determination of the fetal sex may be performed when an X-linked condition is present in a family, e.g. Simpson–Golabi–Behmel syndrome (septal defects, pulmonary stenosis, coarctation, TGA):
  - No confirmatory invasive test is offered as the accuracy is high, although not 100%.

Fetal electrocardiography

- Theoretically valuable in determining rhythm and myocardial health.
- Only available in a small number of centres at present.
- Requires expensive technology.
- Not used in routine clinical practice.

Fetal magnetic resonance imaging

Introduction

Fetal MRI:

- is safe beyond the 1st trimester when performed within internationally accepted energy limits
- is now an established imaging adjunct for many static organs, particularly the fetal brain
- of the heart has long been limited by:
    - structure size
    - fast heart rate
    - lack of external cardiac gating
    - uncontrolled fetal movement
    - cardiovascular fetal MRI is now rapidly developing.

Standard MRI sequences

Certain standard MRI sequences may currently be of value in cases where ultrasound is limited or important aspects of diagnosis cannot be resolved by echocardiography alone.

Single-shot fast spin echo (SSFSE) sequences

T2-weighted sequences offer 'black blood'-like contrast which may offer useful imaging of the extracardiac vasculature. These sequences have a short acquisition time and are generally more robust to minor fetal movements.

Balanced steady-state free precession (bSSFP) sequences

These 'bright blood' sequences produce good contrast between the blood pool and surrounding tissue. They can be useful for assessing intracardiac structures as well as the extracardiac vasculature; however, they are more susceptible to motion artefacts. When combined with SSFSE sequences, tissue characterization (e.g. of intracardiac tumours) may also be possible.

Novel techniques

While not routinely available in a clinical setting, novel MRI techniques may offer a more comprehensive means of assessing the fetal cardiovascular system.

Phase contrast imaging

Retrospective cine gating techniques can allow for estimation of flow rates in the major fetal vessels. These are currently limited to a research setting. Similar techniques have allowed for estimation of intravascular oxygen content in late gestation fetuses.

Spatiotemporal motion correction

Motion-corrected 2D–3D registration techniques offer the potential to provide highly detailed 3D information for static structures, such as the major vessels.

Summary

A clear clinical role of fetal cardiovascular MRI is yet to be established. Newer MRI techniques offer the possibility of generating comprehensive fetal cardiovascular anatomy, function, and haemodynamic information, comparable to cardiac MRI studies in postnatal life.

Chapter 9

Structural abnormalities

Introduction

This chapter gives an overview of the classification of structural cardiac anomalies used in the detailed description and discussion in the following chapters. These fundamental points apply throughout:

- It is essential to begin by establishing the left and right sides of the fetus before going on to define the morphological features of each chamber and vessel and to demonstrate the cardiac connections (➲ Chapters 4 and 6).
- Structural cardiac anomalies will be classified according to the segmental approach to cardiac anatomy (see ➲ Chapter 4).
- There may be more than one cardiac abnormality present, thus the initial scan should be full and detailed.
- There are limitations to the detail that can be obtained prenatally even in technically excellent scans because:
  - fetal size in early gestation may limit resolution
  - some lesions evolve *in utero*
  - postnatal changes alter haemodynamics.
- Having found a cardiac anomaly, a detailed search for non-cardiac conditions is indicated in order to allow as accurate counselling and management planning as possible.
- Some structural anomalies can be or have been considered variations of normal; the distinction between normal and abnormal is not always clear cut and may depend as much on the context or other features (associations, cardiac or otherwise) as on the anatomy alone. Examples of such include:
  - TR in early gestation
  - complete situs inversus with dextrocardia
  - right aortic arch (➲ pp. 101–2)
  - aberrant origin of a subclavian artery (➲ pp. 102–4)
  - bilateral or single left-sided SVC (➲ p. 87).
- These anatomical findings are discussed at various points as relevant.

Classification of structural congenital heart disease

Left-sided structural cardiac anomalies

See ➲ Chapter 10.

Venoatrial

- Partial anomalous pulmonary venous drainage
- Total anomalous pulmonary venous drainage
- Left-sided SVC.

Atrioventricular

- Mitral atresia (absent left AV connection)
- Mitral hypoplasia.

Ventricular-arterial

- Aortic stenosis
- Aortic atresia
- Hypoplastic left heart syndrome.

Arterial

- Coarctation of the aorta
- Interrupted aortic arch
- Right aortic arch
- Aberrant subclavian artery.

Right-sided structural cardiac anomalies

See ➲ Chapter 11.

Venoatrial

- Inferior and superior venae cavae
- Azygous/hemiazygous connections.

Atrioventricular

- Tricuspid atresia (absent right AV connection)
- Ebstein's anomaly/tricuspid valve dysplasia.

Ventricular-arterial

- Pulmonary stenosis
- Pulmonary atresia with intact septum
- Tetralogy of Fallot
- Tetralogy with absent pulmonary valve
- Pulmonary atresia with VSD
- DORV.

Septal abnormalities

See ➲ Chapter 12.

Atrial septal defect

- Secundum
- Sinus venosus type
- (Primum ASD—see ➲ Partial AVSD).

Ventricular septal defect

- Perimembranous
- Inlet
- Outlet
- Muscular (with more detailed description of location if possible).

Atrioventricular septal defect

- Partial
- Complete
- Intermediate type.

Abnormal ventriculoarterial connections

See ➔ Chapter 13.

- Transposition of the great arteries
- Congenitally corrected transposition of the great arteries
- Common arterial trunk.

Miscellaneous lesions

See ➔ Chapter 14.

- Double inlet left ventricle
- Isomeric anomalies.

Detailed consideration of anomalies

- The following chapters in this handbook explain these lesions and describe the:
  - incidence (mainly based on postnatal figures)
  - anatomy
  - associated cardiac anomalies
  - haemodynamics when appropriate
  - ultrasound features and evolution *in utero*
  - non-cardiac associations.
- An account of the postnatal options and course of the cardiac lesions is given particularly when fetal findings or management may be relevant to these.

Chapter 10

Left-sided abnormalities

Venoatrial junction

Partial anomalous pulmonary venous drainage (pAPVD)

Incidence

- <1% of CHD.

Anatomy

- 1 or more of the 4 pulmonary veins, more frequently right sided, drain somewhere other than the left atrium:
  - most commonly into the right atrium
  - but otherwise IVC, SVC, left innominate vein, or coronary sinus.
- There may be abnormal pulmonary arterial supply (as in Scimitar syndrome).

Associated cardiac anomalies

- ASD most common.
- Any other can occur.
- May be isolated.

Prenatal significance

- Since pulmonary blood flow is small in the fetus:
  - it is difficult to diagnose
  - there is no haemodynamic significance in the absence of severe stenosis of the vein(s).

Ultrasound (U/S) features

- Very hard to diagnose on imaging unless other abnormalities raise suspicion as in:
  - left atrial isomerism suspected (➔ Chapter 14)
  - abnormal heart position (usually rightward displacement)
  - abnormal pulmonary arterial imaging with one (usually the right) being much smaller
  - abnormal source of pulmonary blood flow identified from descending aorta
  - superior sinus venosus ASD
  - Doppler indicates an obstructed pulmonary venous waveform.

Non-cardiac associations

- Pulmonary hypoplasia.

Postnatal implications

- Altered haemodynamics are determined by:
  - the number of pulmonary veins involved
  - the presence or absence of stenosis of the vein(s).
- Surgery to correct may be indicated but is not always required or practicable if the lesion is isolated and unobstructed.

Total anomalous pulmonary venous drainage (TAPVD)

Incidence

- Approximately 1% of CHD with male:female ratio of 4:1.

Anatomy

There is no direct communication between the pulmonary veins and the left atrium; categories are defined by drainage site:

- Supracardiac (50%): the pulmonary venous confluence drains into the right SVC either directly or via a left vertical vein and left innominate vein.
- Cardiac (20%): the pulmonary veins drain either directly into the right atrium or through a confluence into the coronary sinus.
- Infracardiac/infradiaphagmatic (20%): the pulmonary venous confluence drains either to the portal vein, ductus venosus, hepatic vein, or IVC.
- Mixed (10%): a combination of these variations.

Associated cardiac anomalies

- A feature of complex CHD as seen in atrial isomerism (➔ Chapter 14) in which both pulmonary venous configuration and any associated obstruction have an important impact on management strategies
- Hypoplastic left heart (➔ pp. 95–7)

U/S features

- Difficult to detect prenatally in isolation but may be suspected in the context of isomerism
- May be possible to define a confluence behind the left atrium (Fig. 10.1)
- Left-sided structures may be smaller than right and are occasionally hypoplastic
- Doppler interrogation may reveal evidence of one or more sites of obstruction (Fig. 10.2)

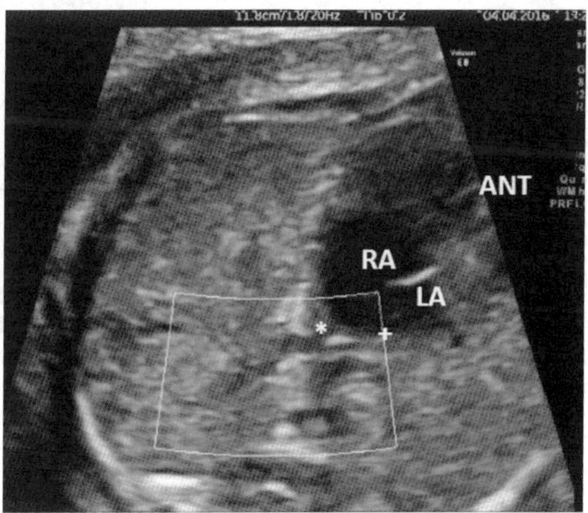

Fig. 10.1 Oblique 4-chamber view showing confluence (*) behind atrial mass with no entry of pulmonary veins to LA.

(a)

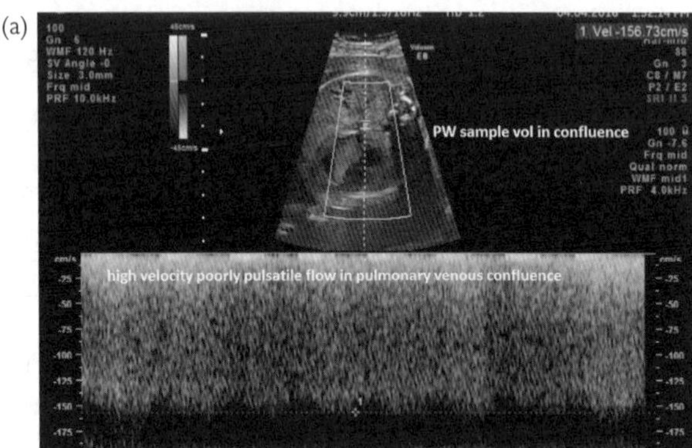

(b)

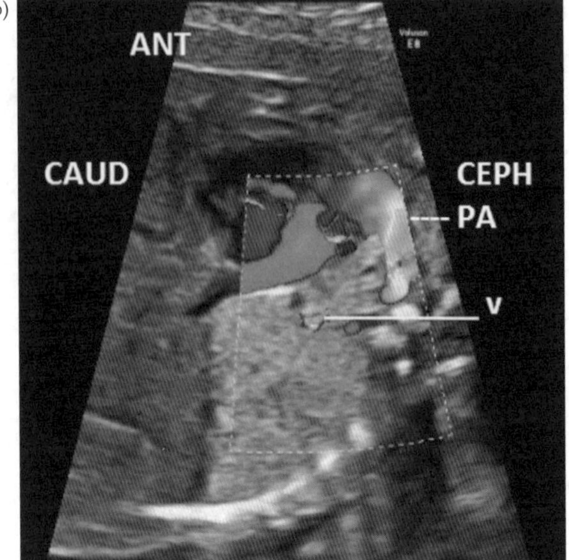

Fig. 10.2 (a) PW Doppler signal in pulmonary venous confluence (v) showing high velocity poorly pulsatile signal indicative of obstruction. (b) Colour flow signal with aliasing in a confluence behind LA. (See colour plate section).

Evolution and prognosis in utero

- Prognosis will be determined by obstruction/hypoplasia of the veins and by other cardiac anatomy.
- Stenosis may not be apparent until after birth and pulmonary blood flow increases.

Associated non-cardiac anomalies

- Isomerism.
- Cat eye syndrome (complex anomaly of chromosome 22).

Postnatal prognosis and management

- Right-to-left shunting at atrial level is required for survival and the fossa ovalis can be, or rapidly become, restrictive.
- The precise anatomy and severity of venous stenosis will define timing for corrective surgery but will be early if veins are obstructed (especially common in infradiaphragmatic form).

Left-sided SVC

See also ➲ Chapter 11.

- Bilateral SVCs may or may not be connected by a innominate/bridging vein.
- This is increasingly identified as 3VT views become part of the routine screening fetal echocardiogram (➲ Chapter 7, p. 64).
- May be recognized *in utero* as it often causes a prominent coronary sinus (Fig. 10.3) which can be a manifestation of other much rarer conditions including left heart hypoplasia and TAPVD to coronary sinus
- Normally an incidental finding of no functional significance but sometimes seen in association with other cardiac anomalies
- Bilateral SVCs can be associated with coarctation (➲ pp. 98–100) but may also accompany ventricular and arterial disproportion (left-sided structures smaller) in the absence of coarctation; the mechanism for this is unclear.

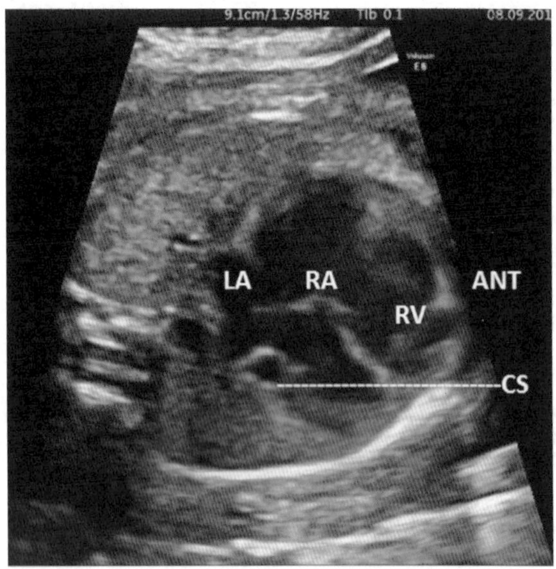

Fig. 10.3 Prominent coronary sinus in 4-chamber view.

Atrioventricular junction

Mitral atresia (absent left AV connection)

Incidence
- A rare anomaly.

Anatomy
- Complete obstruction to flow across mitral valve.

Associated cardiac anomalies
- Part of hypoplastic left heart syndrome (➔ pp. 95–7).
- Or in conjunction with double outlet right ventricle with or without VSD.
- Great arteries may be discordant.
- Coarctation if VSD present and arteries normally connected.
- Pulmonary stenosis/atresia if arteries are transposed.

Haemodynamics
- Dependent on left-to-right flow at atrial level which can become restricted at foramen ovale.
- If an arterial outflow is dependent on VSD:
  - VSD can become restrictive
  - resulting in stenosis or atresia of relevant arterial outlet.

U/S features
- 4-chamber views are abnormal with marked atrial and ventricular disproportion (Fig. 10.4).
- The mitral valve is seen as a small rigid structure with no flow across it demonstrable by Doppler interrogation.
- All left-sided structures small.
- Flow at atrial level will be exclusively left to right (Fig. 10.5).
- Associated lesions should be identified.

Association with non-cardiac anomalies
- Variably reported, no consistent pattern.

Postnatal prognosis and management
- Largely determined by size of LV but rarely suitable for biventricular repair.
- Duct dependency will be determined by associated lesions.

Mitral hypoplasia

- Definition subjective but can be helped by use of Z-scores (obtained from one of the readily available Apps).
- May evolve into atresia/hypoplastic left heart.
- Essentially similar associations and haemodynamic consequences to atresia.
- Valve looks to open on imaging and Doppler may reveal regurgitation more readily than forward flow.
- Occasional overall small left heart without major valvar obstructions remains suitable for biventricular repair (often with coarctation).

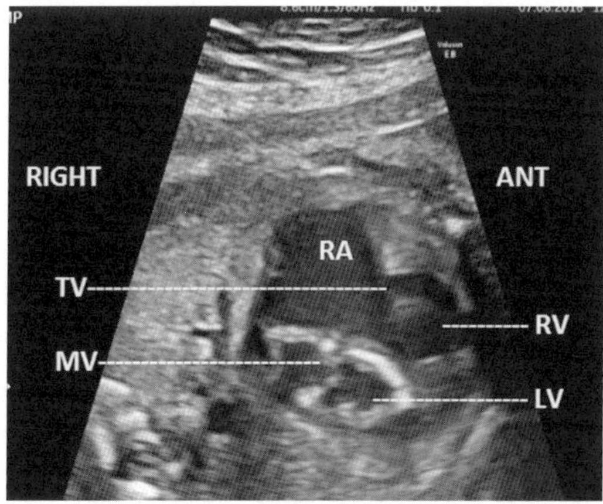

Fig. 10.4 4-chamber view in atrial systole/ventricular diastole. Small MV does not open, TV is fully open. LV cavity is small. Left AV valve atresia ('mitral atresia').

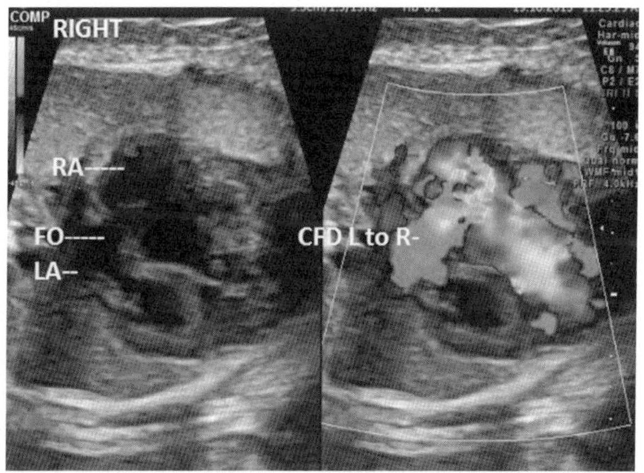

Fig. 10.5 4-chamber view with colour flow Doppler showing L-to-R flow across foramen ovale in left heart obstruction. (See colour plate section).

Ventriculoarterial junction

Aortic stenosis

Types

- Supravalvar:
  - Rarely identified in the fetus.
  - Strongly associated with Williams syndrome.
  - Very rarely autosomal dominant.
- Subvalvar:
  - Often associated with interrupted arch with VSD or more complex anatomy.
  - Often a progressive postnatal finding rather than a fetal diagnosis.
- Valvar:
  - The commonest form present in the fetus and early post-fetal life.

Aortic valve stenosis

Incidence

- 3–6% of CHD with male:female ratio approximately 4:1.
- Severity ranges from mild to severe and often progresses *in utero*.

Associated cardiac anomalies

- Other left-sided lesions including coarctation of the aorta.
- May be part of more complex CHD.

Haemodynamics

- Mild and moderate stenosis can be well tolerated *in utero*.
- Severe stenosis characterized by:
  - LV systolic function reduced
  - LV dilation
  - LV wall hypertrophy
  - progressive mitral regurgitation
  - left-to-right flow can develop at atrial level (bidirectional atrial flow can be a feature in normal hearts at later gestation).
- Left ventricular hypertrophy with progressive cavity obliteration may result in hypoplastic left heart.
- Considered critical if hydrops develops or likely to be duct dependent postnatally.

U/S features of valvar stenosis

- Mild stenosis may be difficult to detect prenatally.
- Valve may look thickened (Fig. 10.6) or doming (i.e. restricted opening of leaflets).
- In more severe cases the valve ring is small.
- There may be post-stenotic dilatation of the ascending aorta.
- If the LV is healthy, blood velocity in the ascending aorta will be increased (Fig. 10.3; ➔ Chapter 6).
- Ascending aortic Doppler velocity falls or becomes normal as LV fails.
- Aortic Doppler waveform reveals retrograde flow in transverse and even ascending aorta if critical.

- LV may appear normal but may become either:
  - dilated with poor contractility (Fig. 10.7) and mitral regurgitation, or
  - hypertrophied with a LV small cavity and reduced contractility.
- Lining of the LV cavity may become bright and echogenic due to development of endocardial fibroelastosis (Fig. 10.8).

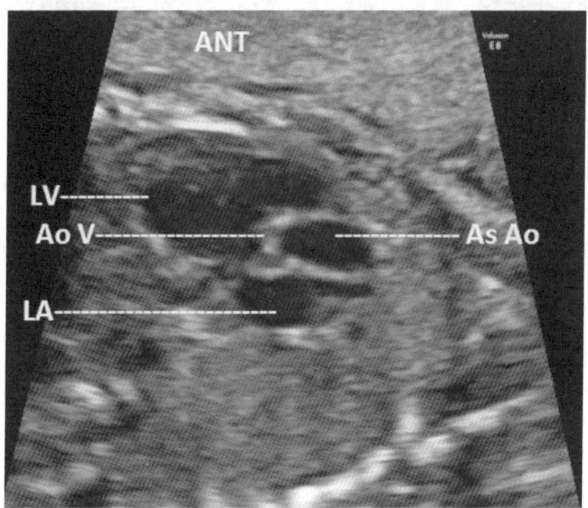

Fig. 10.6 Long axis in ventricular systole showing thick doming and poorly opening AoV.

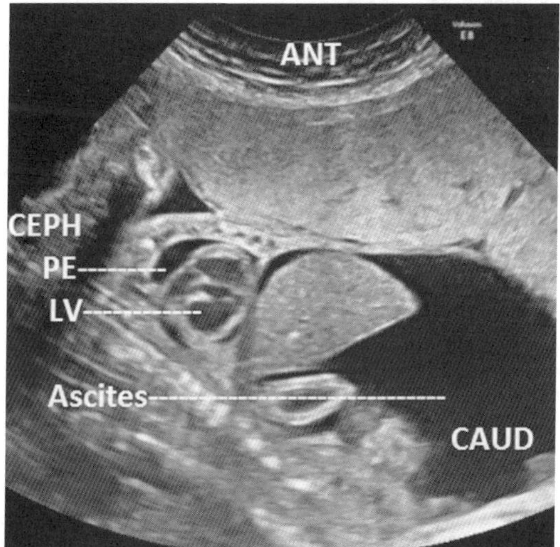

Fig. 10.7 Whole body sagittal section showing dilated LV and evidence of hydrops.

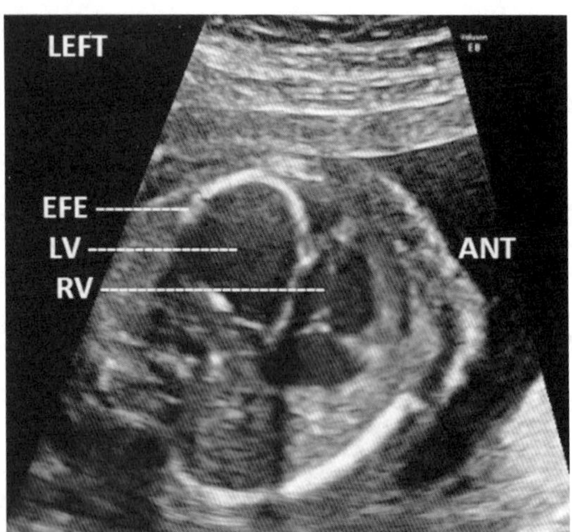

Fig. 10.8 4-chamber view with dilated LV and echobright endocardium indicating endocardial fibroelastosis.

Evolution and prognosis in utero

- This lesion usually progresses during pregnancy.
- In severe and critical AS, hydrops may develop leading to intrauterine death.
- Deterioration in LV function and diminishing LV volume may indicate that a functioning LV may not be achievable postnatally.
- This observation may be a reason to consider:
  - balloon dilatation—this is controversial
  - delivery if a viable gestation has been reached
- The poor prognosis associated with severe AS may justify consideration of an *in utero* procedure to relieve obstruction before LV failure occurs.

Association with non-cardiac anomalies

- Isolated valvar AS has a low association with non-cardiac anomalies although can be associated with syndromes including:
  - Turners syndrome (AS generally commoner in males)
  - Noonan syndrome (rarely).

Postnatal prognosis and management

- Depends on severity of stenosis and LV function.
- If favourable, percutaneous balloon valvuloplasty may provide a good relief of stenosis.
- For others, open surgical valvotomy may be needed.
- Valve replacement is likely in time.
- A few are not suitable for biventricular repair.
- Irreversible and progressive pulmonary vascular disease may give a poor outlook in the long term even if biventricular repair has been achieved early in life.

Aortic atresia

- Usually seen in the context of hypoplastic left heart syndrome (see following topic).

Hypoplastic left heart syndrome

Incidence

- Approximately 1% of structural CHD but represents a higher percentage of cases identified prenatally.

Anatomy

- Variations in precise anatomical phenotype are recognized.
- For classical HLHS, there is both mitral and aortic atresia resulting in a small, diminutive LV (Fig. 10.4) and absence of flow through the left side of the heart.
- In some, left heart structures are significantly hypoplastic in spite of a small amount of flow through both mitral and aortic valves; these cases may be considered as HLHS:
    - Establishing whether a biventricular circulation will be achievable postnatally in these cases can be difficult; if the LV is not apex forming, a 2-ventricular strategy may be unachievable.

Associated cardiac anomalies

- Pulmonary venous drainage is occasionally anomalous.
- All left-sided structures are small including the aortic arch.
- There may be discrete coarctation.
- Rarely a VSD exists and is large enough to result in less severe LV hypoplasia and forward flow through the aortic valve.
- Coronary AV fistulae may occur.

Haemodynamics

- Absence of flow through the mitral valve causes left-to-right shunting through the atrial septum.
- Increased pressure in the left atrium may result in premature closure of the foramen ovale.
- Further increases in left atrial pressure increases pressure in the pulmonary veins with potential irreversible damage to the pulmonary vasculature.
- The LA may decompress through an ascending vein joining the innominate vein (laevo-atrio-cardinal vein).
- Coronary and cerebral perfusion is maintained by retrograde flow from the arterial duct into the aortic arch.

U/S features

- From early in gestation marked disproportion in ventricular size is obvious on the 4-chamber view.
- Left-sided structures may be so small that they are hard to define.
- Lining of the LV may be bright and echogenic due to endocardial fibroelastosis (Fig. 10.8).
- The pulmonary artery is prominent and the aorta threadlike.
- Doppler will demonstrate absent (or minimal) forward flow through both mitral and aortic valves with retrograde flow in the aortic arch (Fig. 10.9).

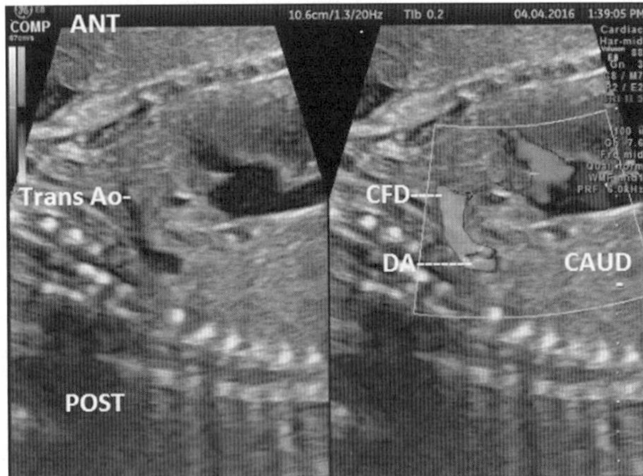

Fig. 10.9 Long-axis view of aortic arch with red colour flow Doppler (CFD) signal indicating flow towards the transducer in the arch, that is to say, retrograde filling from the DA. (See colour plate section).

- Colour Doppler will show entirely left-to-right flow across the atrial septum.
- Some features that suggest less favourable prognosis may be identifiable prenatally including:
  - tricuspid regurgitation, which may be severe
  - abnormal flow pattern in pulmonary veins (➔ Fig. 10.2a)
  - high-velocity (>1 m/s) left-to-right flow across foramen ovale (Fig. 10.10).

Evolution and prognosis in utero

- Usually well tolerated during pregnancy.
- Tends to progress in terms of:
  - hypoplastic but initially patent valves may become atretic
  - foramen ovale may close
  - right ventricular function may become compromised.
- The possibility of further damage to lung vasculature if the atrial septum closes is the rationale for considering an *in utero* procedure to open and then to stent a gap in the atrial septum.

Association with non-cardiac anomalies

- In the majority of cases HLHS is an isolated finding but can be seen in association with some chromosomal anomalies including:
  - Turner syndrome
  - Other less common chromosome anomalies.

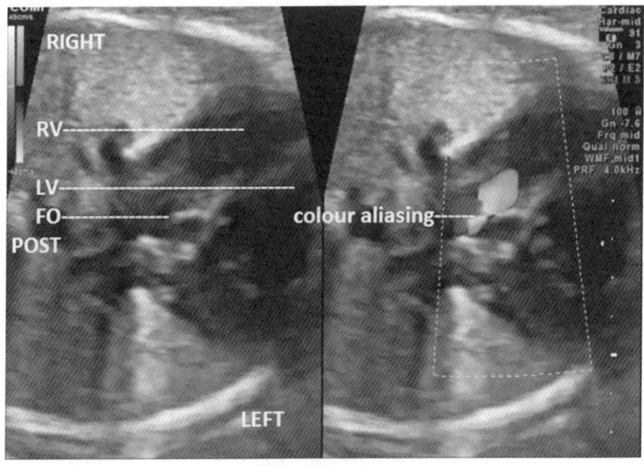

Fig. 10.10 Oblique view of IAS with CFD showing aliasing (i.e. high velocity) in the L-to-R flow across the foramen ovale. Severe left heart obstruction. (See colour plate section).

Postnatal management and prognosis

- Without treatment, death occurs when the arterial duct closes in the first 5–10 days after birth, longer survival is rare.
- Surgical treatment for HLHS is palliative and involves surgery in the early newborn period (the Norwood procedure) and at least 2 further operations during the pre-school period to establish a cavo-pulmonary (Fontan type) circulation but even after this:
  - the chances of reaching school age and beyond is approximately 50% when a decision is made at the time of fetal diagnosis for active post-natal management
  - survival with a good quality of life may be achieved but long-term outcome is still to be fully evaluated.
- Transplantation is an alternative to the Norwood procedure but is rare or impossible in many countries.
- The indications for and validity of opting for palliative care postnatally are matters for ongoing discussion

Arterial abnormalities

Coarctation of the aorta

Incidence

- 8–10% of CHD with male:female ratio approximately 2:1.

Anatomy

- Coarctation of the aorta is recognized in 3 forms depending on age at presentation:
  - neonatal
  - infant
  - adult.
- These may or may not represent a spectrum of the same disease.
- The neonatal form, by virtue of its early presentation, is more likely to have features which can be identified prenatally.
- Narrowing of the aorta, usually distal to the 3rd head and neck vessel (left subclavian artery) and just distal to the aortic isthmus, close to the site of DA attachment to the aorta.

Associated cardiac anomalies

- Associations include:
  - bicuspid aortic valve in up to 85% of cases
  - potential to develop subaortic stenosis
  - VSD in around 25% of cases
  - left SVC is associated.
- Coarctation is also seen in conjunction with complex CHD.

Haemodynamics

- Forward flow through all left-sided valves is present.
- Obstruction from coarctation will not develop until after the arterial duct closes; thus this diagnosis can be suspected but not proven until the postnatal circulation is established.

U/S features

- For those presenting neonatally, significant ventricular and arterial disproportion is usually present by the 20-week anomaly scan (Fig. 10.11).
- PA may be up to twice as big as the aorta.
- 3-vessel view may demonstrate a small transverse aortic arch (Fig. 10.12).
- In the presence of VSD, ventricular disproportion may be less obvious but arterial disproportion will still be present.
- However, it is a difficult diagnosis to make prenatally because:
  - some ventricular disproportion (RV >LV) is normal, especially during the 3rd trimester
  - PA is normally >aorta in 3rd trimester
  - such disproportion is also seen in the presence of a left-sided SVC and an otherwise structurally normal arch and heart
  - arch may look normal whilst DA is patent.

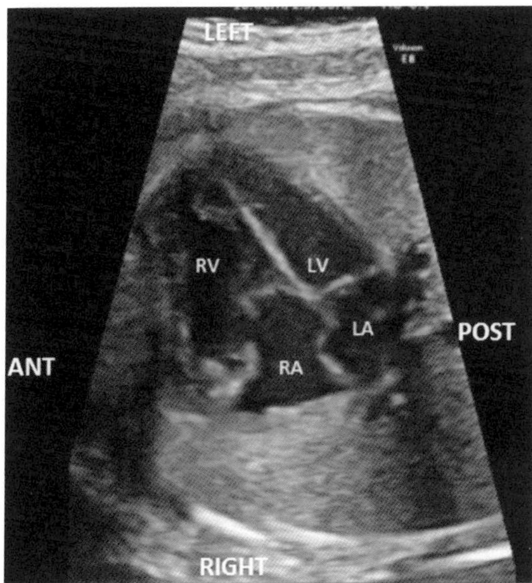

Fig. 10.11 4-chamber view showing disproportion (RV >LV) but both ventricles form the cardiac apex.

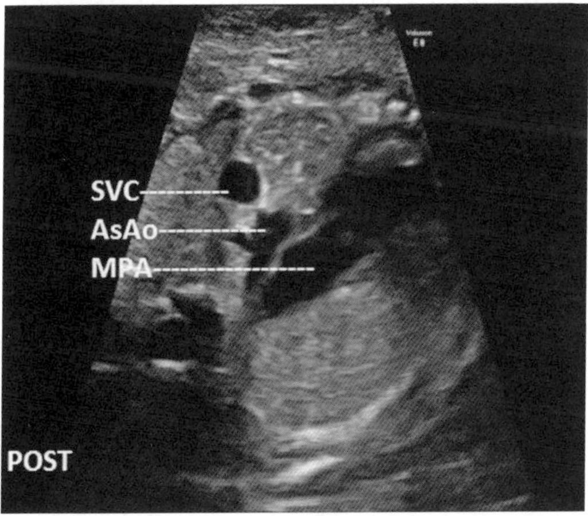

Fig. 10.12 3VT view showing small Ao in likely case of coarctation.

Evolution and prognosis in utero

- This lesion is well tolerated while the duct remains open.
- The features may become more obvious as gestation increases.
- Aortic stenosis may develop in those with an abnormal aortic valve.

Association with non-cardiac anomalies

- Chromosomal anomalies, particularly Turner syndrome:
  - 30% of Turner syndrome have a coarctation but may not present in the neonatal period and therefore not be suspected prenatally.
  - Other rarer chromosome anomalies.

Postnatal prognosis and management

- If the fetal diagnosis is strongly suspected and there may be delay in postnatal cardiology assessment, prostaglandin should be commenced intravenously in the early hours after birth.
- Coarctation presenting in the neonatal period requires surgery with a high success rate; long-term follow-up is appropriate and sometimes a further intervention is required, usually in the form of a transcatheter procedure.

Interrupted aortic arch

Incidence

- 1% of critical neonatal CHD.

Anatomy

- Total interruption of the aortic arch.
- Classification is based on the site of interruption.

Associated cardiac anomalies

- A VSD is usually present.
- The aortic valve is often bicuspid.
- May be seen in association with a common arterial trunk.

Haemodynamics

- Coronary arteries and those head and neck vessels proximal to the interruption will be perfused from the LV.
- Those arch vessels distal to the obstruction will be perfused retrogradely from the arterial duct.
- Blood supply to the lower body is dependent on the presence of an arterial duct.

U/S features

- Essentially similar those seen in coarctation:
  - Ventricular disproportion, RV >LV.
  - Arterial disproportion, PA >aorta.
- A VSD may be visible on 2D imaging and colour Doppler.
- There is often subaortic LV outflow narrowing on imaging.
- Interruption may be visible on imaging:
  - Head and neck vessels proximal to interruption look like fingers heading toward the head (Fig. 10.13).
  - A 'shepherd's crook' pattern of the normal aortic arch cannot be identified.
- Doppler demonstrates retrograde flow to the distal arch from the arterial duct.

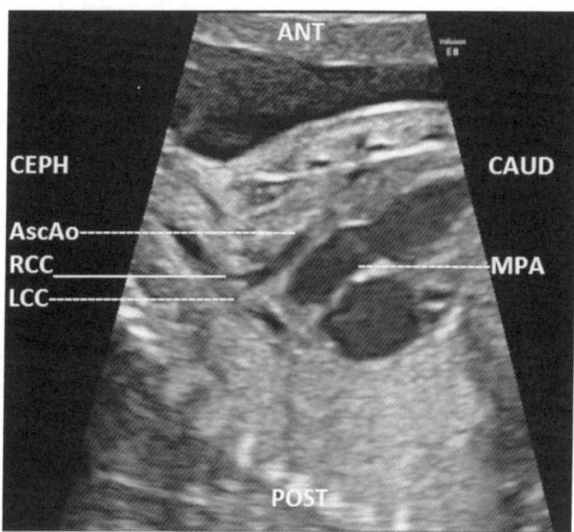

Fig. 10.13 Arch view showing small ascending Ao dividing into 2 head and neck branches (right (RCC) and left common carotid (LCC) arteries) and not continuing into transverse arch. Interrupted aortic arch (there is also TGA in this case).

Evolution in utero

- Usually well tolerated during pregnancy.
- All features may become more obvious as gestation progresses.

Association with non-cardiac anomalies

- Interrupted aortic arch has a strong association with non-cardiac anomalies.
- Particularly associated with 22q11 deletion syndrome.

Postnatal management and prognosis

- Neonatal circulation is duct dependent and tends to be less stable than duct-dependent coarctation.
- Early surgery to repair the arch and close the VSD will be necessary and prognosis is largely defined by the size of the arch, length of interruption, and the presence and nature of any other cardiac anomalies.

Right aortic arch

Incidence

- Probably about 0.5% in situs solitus in a low-risk fetal population.

Anatomy

- Most common mirror image of a left arch.
- Arch shape may vary.
- Branching abnormalities may occur, particularly aberrant right subclavian artery from the descending aorta.
- Coarctation is only rarely described.

Associated cardiac anomalies

- Complete situs inversus with dextrocardia is likely to have right aortic arch.
- Intracardiac anatomy can be normal.
- Any intracardiac anomaly can occur but right aortic arch is particularly highly associated with:
  - tetralogy of Fallot
  - pulmonary atresia with VSD.

Haemodynamics

- Of itself, arch side does not impact fetal haemodynamics.

U/S features

- In 3VT view the aorta is seen to the right of the trachea (Fig. 10.14).
- It can be difficult to distinguish from double/bilateral arch or persistent 5th arch.

Association with non-cardiac anomalies

- May be isolated.
- Reported in association with chromosomal abnormalities even with normal intracardiac anatomy (especially 22q11del).

Postnatal management

- Depends on the full cardiac diagnosis.
- An aberrant left subclavian artery arising distal to the right subclavian artery may cause a symptomatic vascular ring and warrant intervention.

Aberrant subclavian artery

Incidence

- Aberrant right subclavian artery (ARSA) arising from a left aortic arch may occur in up to 2% of individuals.
- Aberrant left subclavian from a right arch is much rarer.

Anatomy

- The right subclavian arises from the proximal descending aorta distal to the left subclavian artery and crosses the mediastinum towards the right:
  - most often behind the oesophagus
  - it can be between oesophagus and trachea
  - or in front of the trachea.

Associated cardiac anomalies

- Commonly there are none.
- Any form of structural CHD can be present.

Haemodynamics

- *In utero* it is very unlikely to be of any significance.
- Postnatally the potential for oesophageal and/or tracheal compression exists depending on coexisting features such as the side and position of the arterial duct or its ligamentous remnant.

U/S features

- Best seen in 3VT view (Fig. 10.15).
- Power Doppler (➔ Chapter 5) confirms low-velocity flow from descending Ao towards right.
- RSA not seen arising from first arch branch (innominate artery).

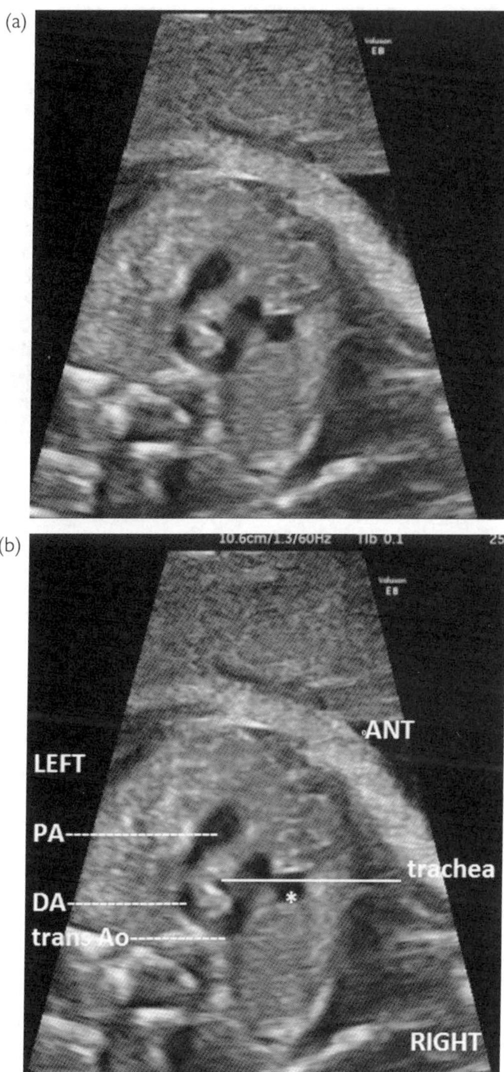

Fig. 10.14 Plain image (a) and annotated (b). 3VT view with right aortic arch passing to right of trachea. * SVC.

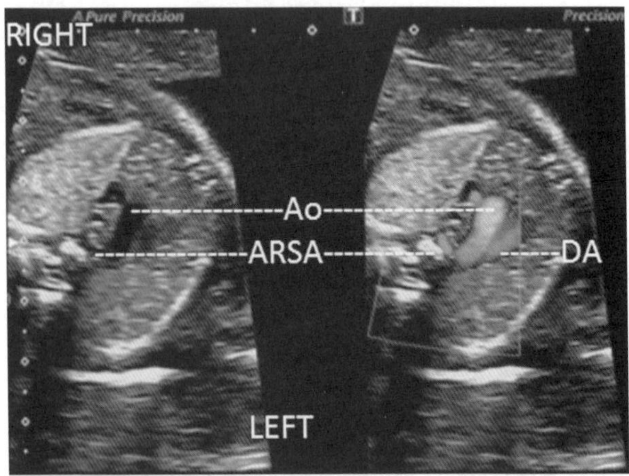

Fig. 10.15 3VT view with left arch and ARSA.

Association with non-cardiac anomalies

- Risk of non-cardiac associations is probably increased and ARSA has been described in trisomy 21 and other syndromes.
- Aberrant left subclavian artery from right arch is strongly associated with 22q11del.

Postnatal management

- Specific management is not necessarily required.
- Surgery is indicated for symptoms or if cardiothoracic surgery is indicated for other lesions and there is a strong risk of oesophageal or tracheal compression.

Double aortic arch

- Incidence unknown.
- May be associated with intracardiac defects or arch abnormalities such as coarctation or interruption.
- Described with oesophageal atresia.
- Incidence of syndromic associations unknown.
- In many series is the commonest symptomatic vascular ring.
- Echocardiographically difficult to distinguish from:
    - right aortic arch with left DA which is much commoner (➲ p. 101)
    - persistent 5th arch (see following topic).
- The ascending aorta divides:
    - A branch goes on each side of the trachea (and oesophagus).
    - Each arch gives off 2 branches.
    - Unless one is interrupted the branches rejoin in the mid thorax
    - The right arch is the larger in at least 70% of cases.

- Unlikely to be of haemodynamic significance *in utero*.
- It is generally thought that symptoms or airway compression is likely in early infancy.
- Thus if suspected will, careful neonatal assessment is indicated.

Persistent fifth aortic arch

- Incidence is unknown, probably very rare.
- Risk of syndromic associations unknown.
- The literature is confusing without universal agreement on the diagnostic criteria.
- To be suspected if any unusual distal ascending aorta branching which does not have characteristics of a double arch or an AP window.
- Is unlikely to matter *in utero*.
- Needs detailed neonatal assessment.

Vascular rings

- Many of the above-mentioned variations/abnormalities in aortic arch side or branching pattern can be associated with compression of the trachea and/or oesophagus, as may distal origin of the LPA (➔ Chapter 11).
- The presence or potential for a clinically significant vascular ring can be hard to predict *in utero* and has been discussed under individual conditions earlier in this section.

Aortopulmonary window

- Rare.
- May be associated with intracardiac or other arch anomalies.
- Rarely associated with syndromes.
- Can occur anywhere from proximal ascending aorta to transverse arch (Fig. 10.16).
- Easily missed on U/S scanning but features include:
  - consistent drop out of signal on image in the same place between aorta and main PA
  - size varies between individuals
  - colour flow Doppler shows low-velocity right-to-left or bidirectional signal.
- Haemodynamically insignificant *in utero* irrespective of defect size.
- Surgery indicated in infancy, timing and details dependent on:
  - size of window
  - other cardiovascular abnormalities present.

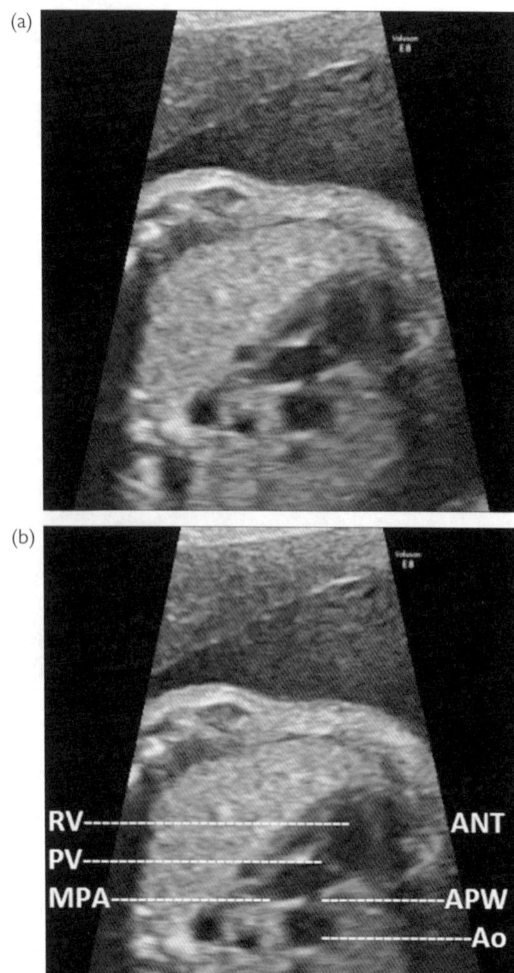

Fig. 10.16 Plain (a) and annotated (b). Oblique view of upper thorax showing aortopulmonary window (APW) between main PA (MPA) and Ao.

Chapter 11

Right-sided abnormalities

Venoatrial junction

Azygous and hemiazygous veins

- Connection between the IVC and SVC territories—azygous vein on the right and hemiazygous on the left in situs solitus—is normal but may be seen echocardiographically.
- Bilateral SVCs are considered a variation of normal, with the left-sided one draining to the RA via the coronary sinus (➔ Chapter 10).

Abnormal systemic venous connections

Incidence

Poorly studied but increasingly detected as echocardiographic screening of low-risk pregnancies becomes more widespread and more detailed.

Spectrum of abnormalities

- Abnormalities of SVC and IVC are rare and are seen:
  - with disorders of laterality (➔ Chapter 14)
  - in sinus venosus type ASDs (rarely recognized in fetal life)—the SVC or IVC (superior and inferior type sinus venosus ASDs respectively) straddle the defect so that blood flows partly into the LA.
- Absence of the portal vein is very rare, the umbilical vein joins directly to the IVC.
- Absent ductus venosus with umbilical vein draining directly to RA:
  - may be associated with cardiac lesions and postnatal persistent pulmonary hypertension
  - is a feature of a number of unusual/rare syndromes and chromosomal abnormalities
  - may be associated with diaphragmatic abnormalities
  - has been reported associated with hydrops.
- Absent ductus venosus with drainage of umbilical vein through the liver (Abernethy malformations):
  - may be associated with postnatal portal hypertension
  - warrants careful postnatal assessment.

Systemic venous anatomy in disorders of laterality

- An interrupted IVC is characteristic of left atrial isomerism. Hepatic veins drain directly to RA and IVC blood flows through the diaphragm, behind the heart to enter the either a right- or left-sided SVC.

U/S features

- Depend on the anatomy present.
- It is important to identify umbilical vein, ductus venosus, and both vena cavae.
- IVC usually does not enter RA:
  - Azygous vein is behind the aorta passing into the thorax (Fig. 11.1)

Associated anatomical features and evolution in utero

- As an isolated anomaly, haemodynamic significance during pregnancy is unlikely.
- The finding should alert to the possible diagnosis of heterotaxy or other conditions mentioned previously.
- Postnatal assessment is appropriate, including defining splenic anatomy/status.

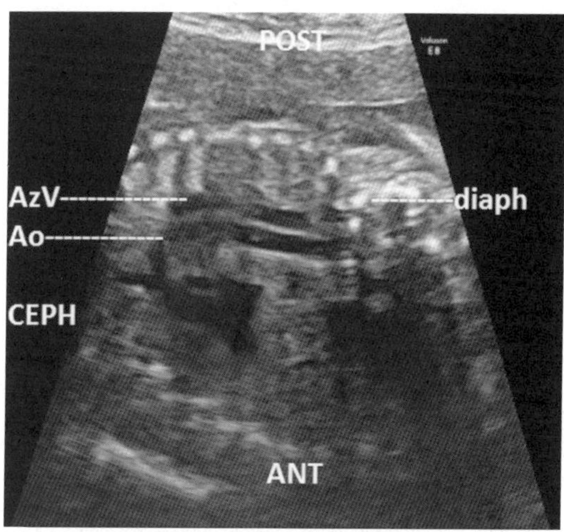

Fig. 11.1 Long-axis view showing vein behind descending aorta as both vessels pass through the diaphragm. Doppler would reveal the nature and direction of flow in each vessel to confirm that the aorta is anterior and that the posterior vessel has flow towards the heart. The vein is to the left of the spine (ascertained in other views) and is therefore strictly a hemiazygos vein. Diaph = diaphragm.

Atrioventricular junction

Tricuspid atresia

Incidence

- 1–3% of CHD.

Anatomy

- The TV is absent and represented by a bar of tissue.
- Also referred to as 'absent right atrioventricular connection'.

Associated cardiac anomalies

- In up to 30% of cases the great arteries are transposed.
- Presence of a VSD is essential for RV filling; postnatally an ASD is needed for survival.
- When the great arteries are normally connected, the pulmonary artery may be small and pulmonary stenosis may be present.
- When the arteries are transposed, the aorta may be underdeveloped with the potential for coarctation to develop postnatally.

Haemodynamics

- In the absence of flow through the TV, blood entering the RA passes through the foramen ovale to LA to LV and enters the RV via the mandatory VSD.
- RV growth will depend on the size of the VSD, as will growth of the artery that arises from this ventricle.

U/S features

- The 4-chamber view is abnormal (Fig. 11.2) with the following features:
  - Small RV.
  - Absent/immobile right AV valve.
  - VSD.
- Extended views will demonstrate:
  - any restriction of flow through foramen ovale (rare)
  - great artery connections
  - relative size of arteries.
- Colour Doppler will confirm direction and velocity of flow.
- Flow in the ductus venosus may be abnormal with retrograde flow during atrial systole:
  - This is not of significance as an indicator of fetal well-being.

Evolution and prognosis in utero

- Altered haemodynamics do not usually cause problems *in utero*.
- Restricted growth of RV and its corresponding artery is more likely if the VSD is small.
- Serial assessment of the smaller artery is appropriate to establish the likelihood of neonatal duct dependency.

Association with non-cardiac anomalies

- Tricuspid atresia is usually an isolated lesion with a low association with either karyotype or syndromal anomalies.
- Cases associated with trisomies have been reported.

(a)

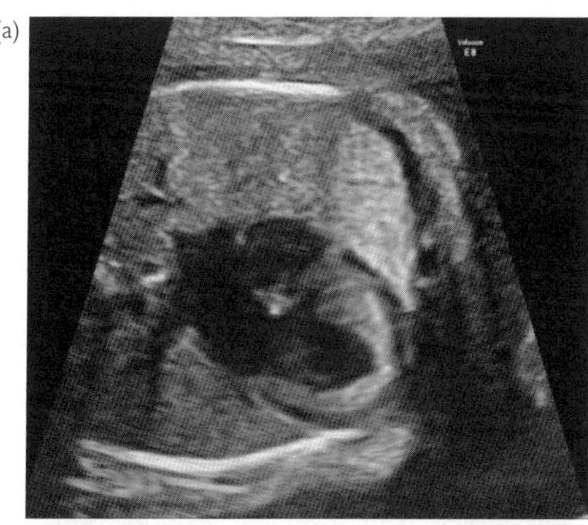

(b)

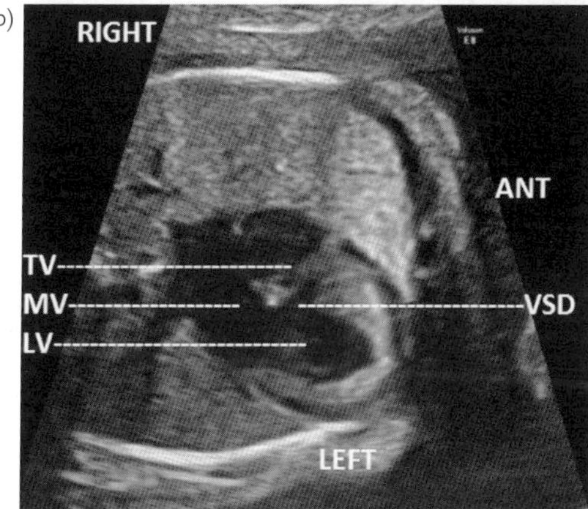

Fig. 11.2 4-chamber view—plain (a) and annotated (b)—in atrial systole showing an open MV, no patent TV, a VSD, and small non-apex-forming RV.

Postnatal prognosis and management

- In cases where RV growth is severely restricted:
  - may be duct dependent
  - neonatal intervention may be required to secure pulmonary blood flow or to repair coarctation
  - not suitable for a biventricular repair
  - usually suitable for a Fontan circulation.

Ebstein's malformation and tricuspid valve dysplasia

Incidence

- Ebstein's malformation represents <1% of CHD.
- Tricuspid dysplasia is rare and incidence is unknown.
- Tricuspid regurgitation is seen in the context of presumed viral infections, twin–twin transfusion or constriction of DA is considered a form of dysplasia

Anatomy

- Ebstein's malformation:
  - Septal and posterior leaflets of the TV are attached closer to the apex of the RV and may also be tethered.
  - This causes part of the RV to be incorporated into the RA termed atrialization of the RV.
  - As a result, there is functional RV and TV hypoplasia often associated with RA dilatation.
- Tricuspid valve dysplasia describes abnormal TV leaflets which may be normally positioned but result in similar haemodynamics to those seen in Ebstein's malformation; in practice, it can to be hard to distinguish prenatally.

Associated cardiac anomalies of both lesions

- Dysplasia is usually isolated, Ebstein's anomaly may be so.
- VSD and PS sometimes occur.
- Many cases of pulmonary atresia with intact ventricular septum (➲ pp. 118–20) also have Ebstein's malformation of the tricuspid valve.
- May be seen in association with congenitally corrected TGA (➲ Chapter 13).

Haemodynamics

- Tricuspid regurgitation is much commoner than stenosis.
- The RA may be enlarged.
- Forward flow through the pulmonary valve may diminish to the point of functional pulmonary atresia.
- Pulmonary artery then fills retrogradely from the ductus arteriosus.
- Pulmonary regurgitation may develop, resulting in flow from aorta through DA, PV, and TV to RA
- This is a critical and poorly tolerated situation with hydrops heralding death which can also occur without progressive deterioration in dysplastic valve disease in particular.
- The above-mentioned changes are usually progressive so careful and frequent monitoring through gestation is appropriate.

U/S features

- The 4-chamber view is abnormal (see Fig. 11.3) with:
  - exaggerated off-setting of the AV valves in Ebstein's malformation
  - thickened leaflets in dysplasia
  - dilated RA
  - increased C:T ratio.
- Beware of the normally positioned AV ring which is not at the same level as the valve leaflets but appears like a tricuspid valve.
- Colour Doppler demonstrates degree of tricuspid regurgitation.

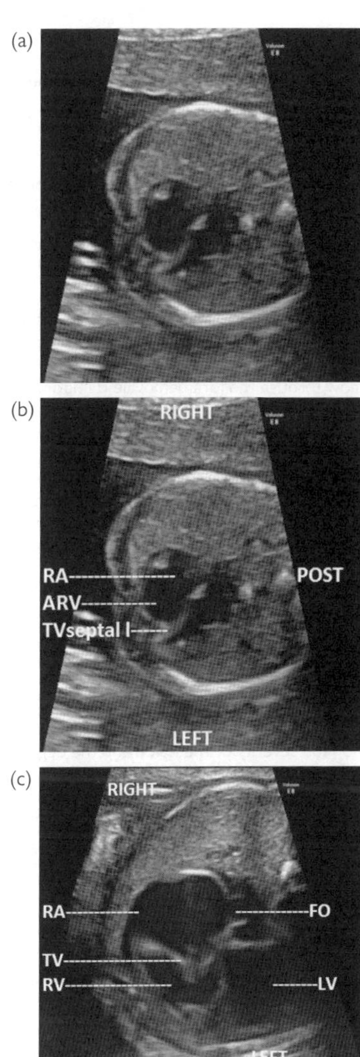

Fig. 11.3 (a) Plain and (b) annotated 4-chamber view of Ebstein's malformation showing marked apical displacement of tricuspid valve septal leaflet (TV septal l). (c) 4-chamber view of dysplastic TV. Thickened leaflets but not displaced.

- Colour Doppler may demonstrate that flow in the pulmonary artery is retrograde.
- Flow in the ductus venosus in atrial systole may become absent or reversed.
- Hydrops may develop.

Evolution and prognosis in utero

- Milder forms of Ebstein's malformation and TV dysplasia may be unrecognized early in pregnancy especially on 2D imaging.
- This lesion tends to progress:
    - TR increases
    - RA enlarges
    - C:T ratio increases
    - Forward flow through the pulmonary artery diminishes
    - Rhythm disturbances—SVT or atrial flutter—may develop as a result of increasing size of RA.
- Unrestricted flow through the foramen ovale is important for fetal (and postnatal) well-being.
- In time, the heart may occupy most of the chest.
- Increasing C:T ratio may compromise lung development.
- Intrauterine death, particularly in the later stages of pregnancy may occur in up to 25% of severe cases and very close monitoring in the 3rd trimester is appropriate.
- Early delivery may be indicated if features of progression and worsening haemodynamics are demonstrated.

Association with non-cardiac anomalies

- Usually an isolated finding but has been reported in association with trisomies or other structural anomalies.
- The association with maternal lithium therapy is recognized but may previously have been overstated.

Postnatal prognosis and management

- This depends on the severity of the lesion and the degree of associated pulmonary hypoplasia.
- In mild to moderate cases, no specific treatment may be needed and the degree of TR may improve as pulmonary vascular resistance falls, enabling increased forward flow through the pulmonary artery.
- In severe cases, options include performing an atrial septostomy and surgery to the TV.
- Mortality for severely cyanosed infants is high.
- Tricuspid dysplasia may improve structurally as well as haemodynamically after birth (or occasionally even before delivery in mild cases or in the context of TTTS (➔ Chapter 23).

Ventriculoarterial junction

Pulmonary stenosis

Incidence
- 5–8% of CHD.

Anatomy
- May be subdivided into:
  - valvar (90%)
  - subvalvar (infundibular)
  - supravalvar
- Valvar PS may be due to dysplastic valve leaflets.
- Subvalvar PS may be due to malalignment of the ventricular septum with VSD.

Associated cardiac anomalies
- PS is often seen as part of more complex CHD.
- Significant pulmonary regurgitation is unusual *in utero* and is usually a manifestation of compromised cardiac function including:
  - tricuspid valve abnormalities
  - constriction of DA.

Haemodynamics
- Mild and moderate PS is usually well tolerated *in utero*.
- Severe PS may cause RV hypertrophy or dysfunction.
- PS can be associated with significant regurgitation:
  - This is particularly seen with a small valve ring and underdeveloped leaflets, termed absent pulmonary valve.
- If there is tricuspid valve abnormality as well, progressive TR can develop.

U/S features
- Milder forms may not be detected *in utero*, especially earlier in pregnancy.
- For moderate and severe forms it may be possible to demonstrate thickened, poorly mobile doming or dysplastic valve leaflets (Fig. 11.4).
- The pulmonary artery may be:
  - smaller than the aorta
  - dilated, particularly with absent pulmonary valve.
- Doppler will demonstrate acceleration across the right ventricular outflow tract, ± a degree of pulmonary regurgitation.
- Flow in the ductus arteriosus will be anterograde but see ➲ p. 116.

Evolution and prognosis in utero
- PS may progress prenatally, possibly even to critical pulmonary stenosis or pulmonary atresia.
- If pulmonary atresia (or severe pulmonary stenosis) develops, flow in the arterial duct becomes retrograde.

Association with non-cardiac anomalies
- Pulmonary stenosis can occur in conjunction with several syndromes including:
  - Noonan's syndrome, Leopard syndrome.
  - Alagille syndrome when the obstruction is usually supravalvar and difficult to identify in the fetus.

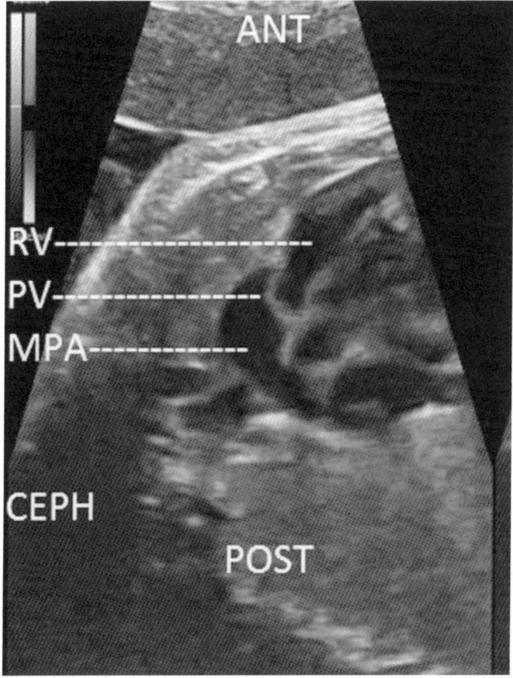

Fig. 11.4 Long-axis view in ventricular systole showing doming, and poorly opening PV.

- Right ventricular outflow tract obstruction is recognized as an acquired form of CHD which may develop in the recipient in TTTS:
  - this may progress even when the TTTS process ceases (with treatment or delivery)
  - there is often RV hypertrophic cardiomyopathy in this setting.

Postnatal prognosis and management

- Type and timing of treatment will be determined by severity and associated cardiac findings.
- Mild isolated forms may regress postnatally.
- If severe:
  - may rarely be duct dependent
  - may require early intervention usually by balloon valvuloplasty.
- Prognosis is determined by:
  - accompanying cardiac abnormalities
  - non-cardiac associations.

Pulmonary atresia with intact ventricular septum (PAIVS)

Incidence

- <1% of CHD.

Anatomy

- The pulmonary valve is atretic represented by a bar of tissue, with no flow across it.
- RV cavity fails to grow normally and may be rudimentary in size.
- Pulmonary artery size is variable.
- Occasionally pulmonary atresia is functional, secondary to severe TR (➔ p. 112).

Associated cardiac anomalies

- In approximately ⅓ of cases, abnormalities of the coronary arteries develop with the following variations:
  - Abnormal origin and distribution.
  - Sinusoidal communications between RV cavity and left or right coronary arteries.
- Coronary arterial anomalies are seen more frequently when the RV is hypoplastic and their presence is a poor prognostic sign.
- The tricuspid valve is rarely completely normal and may show:
  - severe hypoplasia with stenosis
  - Ebstein's malformation.

Haemodynamics

- Flow from the right ventricle can only be retrograde—as tricuspid regurgitation with the potential for right atrial dilatation.
- Some coronary perfusion can be from the RV; this is more adverse postnatally if the aortic diastolic or RV pressures fall after an intervention.
- Lack of forward flow through the right side of the heart results in progressive hypoplasia of RV and sometimes of the pulmonary artery.
- Flow in the arterial duct is retrograde to fill pulmonary artery branches.
- Flow in the ductus venosus may become retrograde in atrial systole.
- Flow across the foramen ovale is increased and non-restrictive flow is important for fetal well-being.

U/S features

- A 4-chamber view of the heart is likely to be abnormal (Fig. 11.5) with a small RV and in some a dilated RA.
- The pulmonary valve will appear as a solid bar of tissue which will show very limited mobility.
- The pulmonary artery may appear relatively normal or may be small, and occasionally hard to define.
- Doppler will demonstrate absence of forward flow across the valve and retrograde flow in the arterial duct (Fig. 11.6).
- Ductal flow appears as forward flow in MPA as it 'bounces' off the atretic valve to pass into pulmonary artery branches.
- Moderate to severe high-velocity TR is usually present.
- Coronary sinusoids may be seen with colour Doppler.

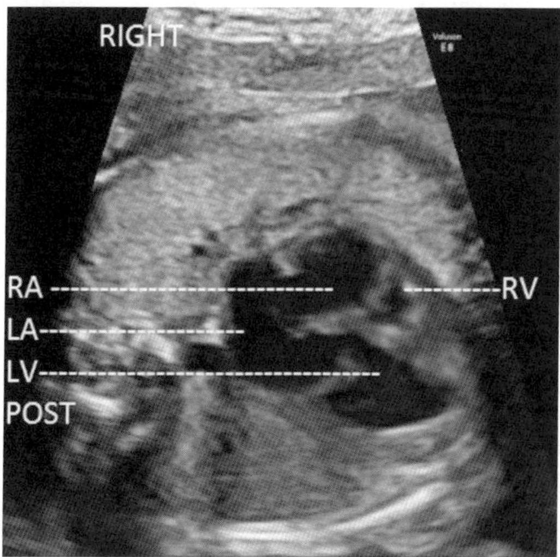

Fig. 11.5 4-chamber view of PAIVS in ventricular systole. The RV cavity is small, the walls are thick, and the IAS bows markedly R to L.

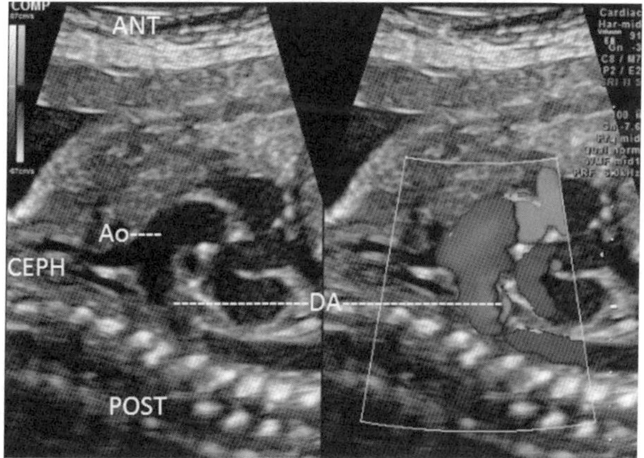

Fig. 11.6 Long-axis view with colour flow Doppler showing retrograde flow in DA in PAIVS. (See colour plate section).

- Secondary/functional atresia should be considered if:
  - the RV cavity is a near normal size
  - the pulmonary artery is a near normal size
  - pulmonary regurgitation is present or develops
  - there is a near normal-sized tricuspid valve with Ebstein's malformation or dysplastic leaflets
  - there is severe TR.

Evolution and prognosis in utero

- This lesion is usually well tolerated *in utero* except in the rare case in which the foramen ovale is severely restrictive.
- Lack of adequate flow through the right side of the heart with progressive RV hypoplasia may prompt consideration of *in utero* intervention to preserve RV growth and function and the possibility of biventricular circulation postnatally

Association with non-cardiac anomalies

- Usually seen in isolation.

Postnatal prognosis and management

- This lesion will be duct dependent.
- The size of the main pulmonary artery and RV will determine the method of intervention.
- Biventricular circulation may be achievable if RV size is adequate.
- Establishing forward flow through the pulmonary valve by radiofrequency ablation and balloon dilatation may allow adequate growth of the RV over time.
- If the RV is considered too small to function, a shunt procedure is performed in the neonatal period as the first step to a Fontan circulation.
- The presence of coronary sinusoids is associated with a risk of sudden death and is considered in some countries as a reason to discuss transplantation rather than conventional interventions.

Tetralogy of Fallot

Incidence

- 10% of CHD.

Anatomy

- Classically consists of 4 anatomical features:
  - VSD in the outlet septum.
  - Subpulmonary stenosis caused by anterior and cephalad deviation of the ventricular septum.
  - Overriding aorta as a consequence of the above-listed features.
  - RV hypertrophy (less obvious in the fetus).

Associated cardiac anomalies

- If the aortic override is >50% into the right ventricle, the lesion is described as double outlet right ventricle (tetralogy type—see ➲ pp. 123).
- Branch pulmonary arteries may be small.
- May be associated with a right-sided aortic arch.
- A small pulmonary valve ring with dysplastic leaflets may be associated with large central PAs; this is termed absent pulmonary valve (➲ pp. 122–3).
- Complete AVSD may accompany tetralogy.

Haemodynamics

- Unrestricted flow into the aorta from both ventricles allows the aorta to grow well.
- Flow into the pulmonary artery may be restricted to a variable degree and growth of the pulmonary artery may be compromised.

U/S features

- The 4-chamber view may be normal although often the cardiac axis is shifted leftwards.
- Extended views will demonstrate (Fig. 11.7):
  - outlet VSD
  - aortic override
  - arterial disproportion (which can be subtle).
- Doppler may demonstrate increased blood velocity through the right ventricular outflow tract and flow into aorta from both ventricles.
- The aortic arch is right sided in about 20% (Fig. 11.7e).
- There may be aortopulmonary collaterals from the aortic arch/descending aorta supplying some pulmonary blood flow.
- Pulmonary regurgitation and large pulmonary arteries are features of the absent pulmonary valve variant (➲ pp. 122–3).

Evolution and prognosis in utero

- Arterial disproportion tends to progress as the right ventricular outflow obstruction becomes more significant.
- The lesion is well tolerated in pregnancy and unlikely to cause fetal compromise.
- Right ventricular outflow tract obstruction may progress to pulmonary atresia.

Association with non-cardiac anomalies

- Tetralogy has a strong association with non-cardiac anomalies.
- Chromosomal anomalies include:
  - trisomy 21
  - trisomy 18
  - trisomy 13
  - 22q11 deletion
  - other rarer anomalies.
- Syndromic with a recognized association include:
  - VACTERL association
  - Alagille syndrome
  - CHARGE association
- Also associated with non-cardiac structural anomalies where no specific syndrome has been defined.

Postnatal prognosis and management

- Postnatal events are largely defined by the degree of right ventricular outflow tract obstruction.
- Only a minority are duct dependent.
- Surgery for correction usually takes place during the first 6 months.
- A few cases have a systemic-to-pulmonary shunt as the first procedure.

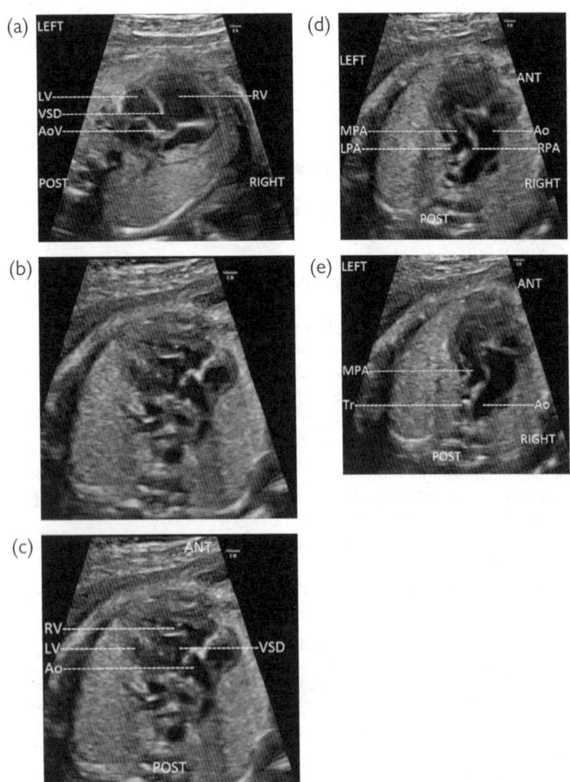

Fig. 11.7 (a) Extended 4-chamber view of tetralogy of Fallot showing VSD with overriding great artery shown on other views to be Ao. (b and c) Outlet view of tetralogy of Fallot—plain (b) and annotated (c)—of same case as (a) showing VSD and overriding aorta. (d) Cephalad inclination of outlet view in tetralogy of Fallot showing main PA approx. 50% diameter of Ao, PAs are confluent. (e) Same case a few frames further on than (c) showing Ao to right of trachea—tetralogy of Fallot with right aortic arch.

Tetralogy with absent pulmonary valve (APV)

- Approximately 2% of cases of tetralogy of Fallot.
- Pulmonary valve ring is small and leaflets are rudimentary and dysplastic (or even absent), producing both pulmonary stenosis and severe pulmonary regurgitation (Fig. 11.8a–c).
- Main pulmonary artery and pulmonary artery branches are usually severely dilated causing compression of developing proximal airways (Fig. 11.8d).
- The VSD is outlet in position as in tetralogy of Fallot.

- 4-chamber view is usually abnormal with RV bigger than LV.
- Colour and pulsed wave Doppler demonstrate to-and-fro flow across the right ventricular outflow tract with both the acceleration of stenosis and regurgitation into RV (Fig. 11.8b, c, e).
- A ductus arteriosus is usually absent.
- Strongly associated with other anomalies particularly 22q11 deletion in at least 25%.
- Less frequently a similar pulmonary valve anatomy is seen in association with an intact ventricular septum when:
  - there is usually a ductus arteriosus
  - pulmonary arteries may not be as dilated.
- *In utero*, pulmonary regurgitation with RV dilatation may increase and arteries become more dilated.
- Death in the neonatal period occurs in up to ⅓.
- Early correction of the anatomy is the aim but prognosis is mainly determined by the degree of airway compromise.

Pulmonary atresia with VSD

- 1:10,000 live births.
- Some are essentially severe tetralogy.
- There is no connection between RV and PA, thus pulmonary blood flow is either:
  - retrograde through the arterial duct which may be in an unusual position, or
  - via collateral arteries arising directly from the aorta—major aortopulmonary communicating arteries (MAPCAs).
- Pulmonary artery branches may be normal, rudimentary, or absent.
- MAPCAs may be identified using colour Doppler:
  - Number is variable.
  - Usually arising from descending aorta distal to the arch.
  - Occasionally arising from transverse aorta or head and neck branches.
  - Can be hard to differentiate from DA.
  - MAPCA anatomy can be difficult to define accurately in the fetus although it has major implications for postnatal management.
- Differential diagnosis includes common arterial trunk which can be hard to distinguish prenatally.
- May be seen in association with:
  - karyotype anomalies, in particular 22q11 deletion
  - other non-cardiac structural anomalies.

Double outlet right ventricle

- Refers to the situation when at least 50% of both arteries arise from RV.
- Major subgroups are:
  - without VSD—usually with left AV valve atresia (➔ p. 90)
  - with subaortic VSD and PS—haemodynamics as in tetralogy or pulmonary atresia VSD (➔ pp. 120–1)
  - with subaortic VSD without PS—haemodynamics like VSD (➔ Chapter 12)
  - with subpulmonary VSD—haemodynamics like transposition with VSD (➔ Chapter 13)
  - with VSD situated away from arterial valves (rarest form).

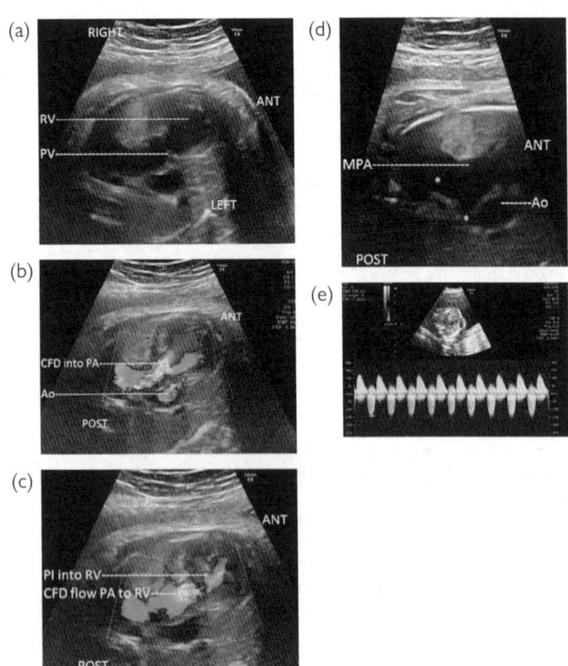

Fig. 11.8 (a) Outlet view in systole showing thickened rigid PV and large main PA (MPA). Tetralogy of Fallot with APV. (b) Same view using colour flow Doppler in ventricular systole showing forward flow RV to PA with some acceleration across PV. (See colour plate section). (c) Same view with colour flow Doppler in ventricular diastole showing PA to RV flow, marked PI in tetralogy of Fallot with APV. (See colour plate section). (d) Huge dilatation of MPA and branches (*) in tetralogy of Fallot with APV. (e) CW Doppler across PV in tetralogy of Fallot with APV showing to and fro signal (+ventricular diastole, −systole)

Arterial abnormalities

- Supravalvar stenosis in MPA is occasionally an isolated lesion.
- More commonly, discrete stenoses or hypoplasia is at the PA bifurcation or beyond:
  - May not be detectable in the fetus even if severe.
  - May be associated with intracardiac abnormalities particularly tetralogy of Fallot and pAVSD.
  - May be associated with syndromes including Williams and Alagille syndromes.
- Distal origin of LPA from the RPA:
  - May be associated with other cardiac abnormalities.
  - Results in LPA forming a sling around the trachea.
  - May be associated with tracheal compression as well as with additional tracheal/bronchial stenosis or even atresia.
  - Is a form of vascular ring (➲ Chapter 10).
- Alternative/additional sources of pulmonary arterial supply from the aorta is a feature of a number of conditions including:
  - Tetralogy of Fallot and pAVSD
  - sequestrated lobe of lung
  - Scimitar syndrome.
- Such arterial vessels can be detected by imaging and Doppler although they may be difficult to delineate accurately in the fetus.

Chapter 12

Septal anomalies

Atrial septal defect

Introduction

- The presence of a patent foramen ovale is essential for right-to-left flow of oxygenated blood returning from the placenta to reach vital organs.
- Distinguishing between a patent foramen ovale and an ASD is difficult and the diagnosis can only be made with certainty if the atrial septum is virtually absent. It is suggested that if the size of the gap in the atrial septum is greater than the diameter of the ascending aorta, then the possibility of a significant ASD postnatally should be considered.
- Atrial shunting is particularly important in some structural cardiac anomalies, particularly those affecting the AV junction, e.g. tricuspid or mitral atresia (➲ Chapters 10 and 11). Restriction to flow at the foramen level may have profound haemodynamic consequences leading to fetal hydrops and intrauterine death.
- In some fetuses, the flap valve of the atrial septum is prominent and appears to have redundant tissue moving into both atria; this is not an abnormal finding but may be associated with an increased incidence of atrial ectopic beats.

Ostium secundum ASD

Incidence

- 10% postnatal CHD but rarely diagnosed *in utero* (see 'Introduction').
- ASD is occasionally an autosomal dominant (often with a long PR interval).

Anatomy

- Defect in fossa ovalis, usually indistinguishable from foramen ovale (see 'Introduction')

Associated cardiac anomalies

- Any structural heart lesion.

Ultrasound features

- Defect in fossa ovalis on 4-chamber view.

Non-cardiac associations

- Holt–Oram syndrome (➲ Chapter 2).

Postnatal prognosis

- Not usually haemodynamically significant for several years; if spontaneous resolution has not taken place by 3–4 years, closure, often by a transcatheter procedure, is performed.

Sinus venosus type ASD

- These are adjacent to either the SVC/RA junction or more rarely the IVC/RA junction.
- The SVC and right upper pulmonary vein straddle the defect in the superior type.
- They are very rarely identified as isolated lesions in the fetus.

Ostium primum ASD

This lesion is more correctly described as a partial atrioventricular septal defect (➲ p. 136).

Ventricular septal defect

Introduction

- VSDs are the most common form of structural cardiac anomaly representing up to 25% of cases of CHD.
- VSDs can be:
  - single or multiple
  - different sizes
  - in different positions
  - isolated, or
  - in association with other forms of CHD.
- These factors influence:
  - prenatal detection rate
  - fetal and postnatal haemodynamic significance
  - likelihood for spontaneous closure.
- VSDs are classified according to their position or relationship to adjacent valves.
- In practice, definition is often not clear cut, frequently with a degree of anatomical overlap.
- For the purposes of fetal diagnosis, VSDs can be classified as follows:
  - perimembranous VSD—commonest
  - inlet muscular VSD
  - outlet muscular VSD
  - muscular VSD—mid and apical
  - doubly committed subarterial.

Anatomy

- The membranous part of the ventricular septum:
  - Small fibrous area in continuity with both tricuspid and aortic valves.
  - In practice, the VSD usually extends into the surrounding muscular septum—hence 'perimembranous' VSD.
- The inlet septum:
  - Lies between the inlet valves—mitral and tricuspid.
  - Posterior to the perimembranous area.
  - Is the part of septum seen on a standard 4-chamber view.
- The outlet septum:
  - Lies just below the aortic valve.
  - In the area where 2 great arteries cross.
  - Anterior to the inlet area.
  - Enables deviation of the ventricular septum and thus the potential to cause narrowing of either outflow tract (deviation or malalignment).
- The remainder of the septum can be described as muscular and subdivided into midmuscular or apical. VSDs here:
  - are frequently multiple
  - can be tiny, or
  - so big that the ventricular septum is virtually absent and there is effectively a single ventricle, or
  - somewhere between these sizes.

- Doubly committed VSDs are:
  - much more common in the Far East than in the West
  - associated with both arterial valves being at the same level and adjacent.

Associated cardiac anomalies

- Found in combination with most cardiac anomalies.
- Perimembranous VSDs are seen in association with:
  - coarctation of the aorta
  - TGA.
- Inlet VSDs may be part of intermediate or complete AVSD.
- Outlet VSDs are an integral part of:
  - tetralogy of Fallot
  - double outlet right ventricle
  - common arterial trunk.
- Muscular VSDs can be seen in combination with most structural cardiac anomalies.

Haemodynamics

- Prenatally VSDs are haemodynamically less important as the 2 sides of the heart function at equal pressures.
- Flow is usually low-velocity right to left in the absence of LV outflow obstruction.
- In some lesions (e.g. tricuspid atresia, mitral atresia, and double inlet left ventricle), a VSD is the only route for blood to enter one of the ventricles.

U/S features

- Small VSDs may be overlooked prenatally on both imaging and by Doppler assessment.
- Artefactual 'dropout' on imaging may be misleading, thus the need to confirm a VSD in different views.
- Perimembranous VSDs (Fig. 12.1):
  - Particularly elusive if small.
  - May have tricuspid valve tissue around defect which will not protrude into the RV as it does postnatally.
  - Colour Doppler may confirm the defect.
- Inlet VSDs:
  - Usually big.
  - No offsetting of AV valves (Fig. 12.2).
- Outlet VSDs:
  - Usually big.
  - Loss of continuity from septum to aorta (Figs 11.3 and 11.7).
  - Aorta (or pulmonary artery in transposition) may appear to override the VSD (Fig. 12.3).
- Muscular VSDs:
  - Many can be seen if the ventricular septum is carefully examined (Fig. 12.4).
  - Colour flow Doppler may give a clearer idea of size or reveal defects unsuspected on imaging.

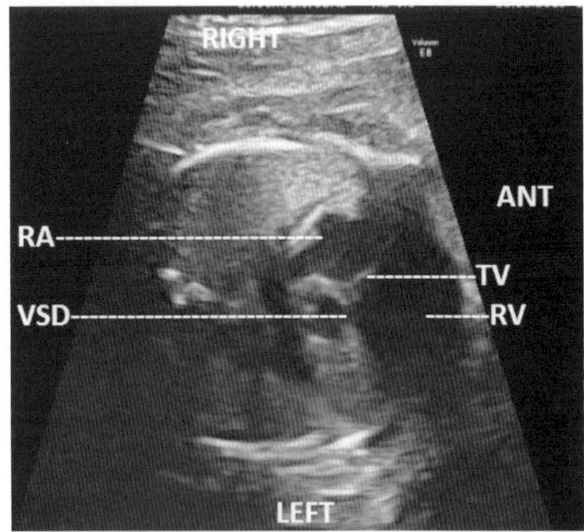

Fig. 12.1 Anterior angulation from 4-chamber view to show perimembranous VSD near aortic outlet and just beneath the septal leaflet of TV.

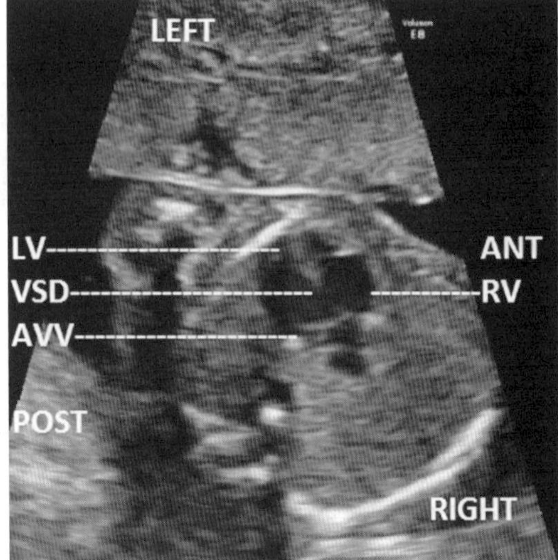

Fig. 12.2 4-chamber view ventricular systole showing closed AV valves without offsetting and a large inlet VSD. Further views in the cycle would show separate AV valve orifices and a normal atrial septum.

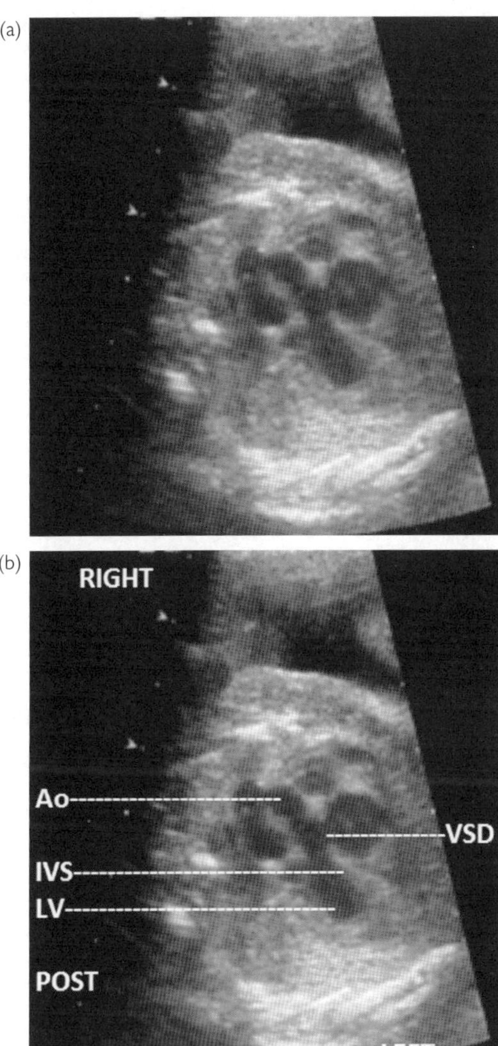

Fig. 12.3 Plain (a) and annotated (b) outlet view showing subaortic VSD with override of the Ao.

- Doubly committed defects are positioned under the leaflets of both arterial valves, being more anterior than either perimembranous or outlet defects. The common postnatal aortic regurgitation is not usually seen.

Evolution and prognosis in utero

- VSDs in isolation are well tolerated in pregnancy.
- Perimembranous and muscular VSDs may close spontaneously in childhood, sometimes even *in utero*.

Associated non-cardiac anomalies

- Inlet VSDs, especially if part of a complete AVSD (➲ p. 136) have a strong association with chromosomal anomalies, particularly trisomy 21.
- Outlet VSDs, in combination with the other recognized cardiac anomalies, are strongly associated with non-cardiac abnormalities, both chromosomal and syndromic, in particular:
    - trisomy 18
    - trisomy 13
    - 22q11 deletion.

Postnatal prognosis and management

- Depends on the haemodynamic status of the VSD which is determined by:
    - size
    - number
    - position
    - presence of other anomalies.
- For larger defects treatment options include:
    - surgical closure
    - if the VSD is large or there are multiple defects or there are other cardiac or extra cardiac problems, a pulmonary artery band may be placed in early infancy to limit pulmonary blood flow
    - transcatheter device closure is possible for a minority VSDs after infancy.

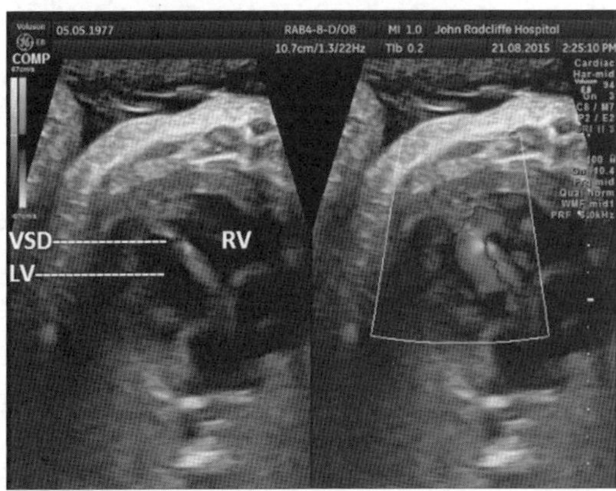

Fig. 12.4 4-chamber view image showing apparently small muscular VSD which with colour flow Doppler is seen to be much larger. The blue Doppler signal reflects flow from RV to LV, the predominant direction in flow for fetal VSD. (See colour plate section).

Atrioventricular septal defects

Introduction

- The atrioventricular septum:
  - is the area identified by offsetting of the atrioventricular valves
  - separates RA from LV (Fig. 4.2).
- Defects affecting this area may be:
  - confined to the atrial portion (partial atrioventricular septal defect, pAVSD), or
  - Involve both the atrial and ventricular portion (complete atrioventricular septal defect, cAVSD).

Partial atrioventricular septal defect

Incidence

- 1–2% of CHD.

Anatomy

- Defect in the primum area of the atrial septum, adjacent and superior to the AV valves.
- Previously referred to as a primum ASD.

Associated cardiac anomalies

- A cleft in the left AV valve is virtually always present.
- Cleft in the tricuspid valve may also be present.
- Abnormalities of the LV outflow tract or coarctation occasionally occur.

U/S features

- 4-chamber view is abnormal with the following features:
  - Loss of offsetting of the AV valves (but still 2 separate AV valves).
  - Defect in the lower part of the atrial septum (Fig. 12.5).
- Doppler may demonstrate flow in this area and often AV valve regurgitation.
- A prominent coronary sinus has a similar 2D appearance but AV valve offsetting will be normal.

Evolution and prognosis in utero

- Well tolerated during pregnancy.
- Severity of AV regurgitation can change in either direction during gestation and in the early newborn period.

Associated non-cardiac anomalies

- May be isolated but also be seen in association with:
  - chromosomal anomalies including trisomy 21 (up to 40%)
  - some structural or syndromic anomalies
  - laterality disorders, especially left atrial isomerism.

Postnatal management and prognosis

- Any neonatal clinical problems are likely to be related to other cardiac or non-cardiac accompaniments.

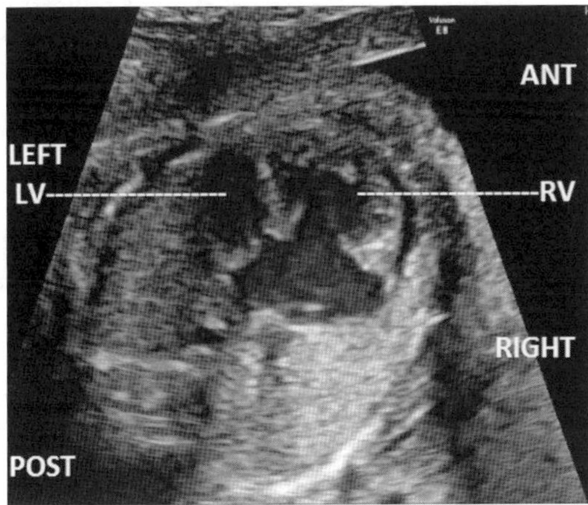

Fig. 12.5 4-chamber view in ventricular diastole showing intact inlet ventricular septum, separate open AV valves, and no atrial septum adjacent to the AV valves: pAVSD.

- Surgery will almost certainly be required to close the defect (± repair of the AV valve); timing is influenced by:
  - associated lesions
  - degree of AV valve regurgitation
  - size of atrial shunt.

Complete atrioventricular septal defect

Incidence

- 2% of CHD.

Anatomy

- Essentially 3 main components of this defect:
  - 'Primum' ASD.
  - Inlet VSD.
  - Single 'common' AV valve.
- Previously described as an endocardial cushion defect.

Associated cardiac anomalies

- May also be seen in association with
  - other VSDs (muscular)
  - tetralogy of Fallot
  - right and left isomerism (➔ Chapter 14).
- May be 'unbalanced' if the common valve is committed more to one ventricle, with the potential for hypoplasia of the other ventricle and the corresponding artery.

U/S features

- The 4-chamber view will be abnormal (Fig. 12.6) with the following features:
  - loss of offsetting of the AV valves
  - functionally single AV valve
  - defect in lower part of atrial septum
  - defect in inlet part of the ventricular septum
  - RV commonly a little larger than LV.
- Doppler may demonstrate regurgitation of the common valve.
- Features of any associated outflow tract abnormalities particularly if ventricles markedly unbalanced.

Evolution and prognosis in utero

- Usually well tolerated although hydrops and intrauterine death is recognized, particularly in the context of an abnormal karyotype.
- A minority of cases develop atrial dysrhythmias.

Association with non-cardiac anomalies

- In 50–75% of cases diagnosed prenatally there is coexistent trisomy 21.
- Also seen in association with trisomies 13 and 18.
- Recognized in the context of other syndromes including VACTERL and CHARGE associations.
- Laterality disorders, particularly right atrial isomerism, usually with severe pulmonary outflow obstruction.

Postnatal management and prognosis

- Corrective surgery usually performed by 6 months of age.

Intermediate type AVSD

This expression is used when the ventricular component is small and there are separate AV valve orifices. Determining the size or even the patency of the ventricular component can be difficult in the fetus.

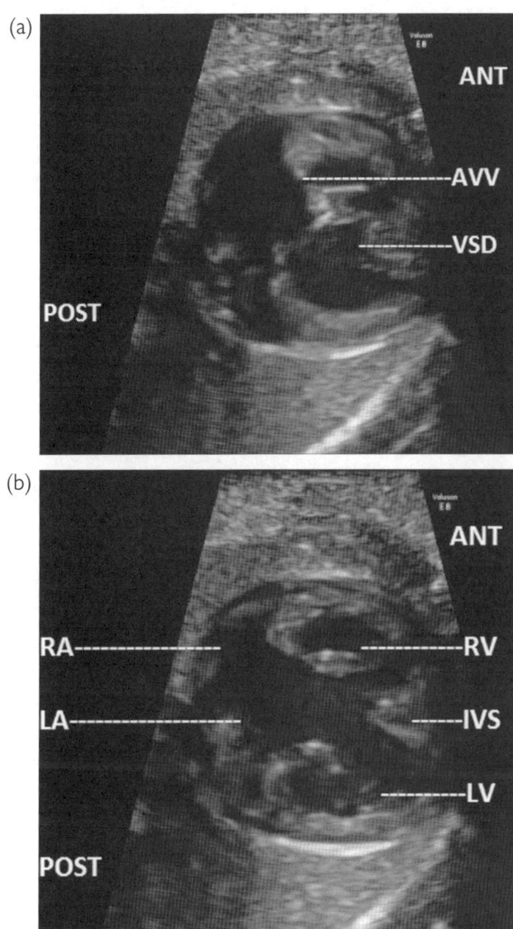

Fig. 12.6 (a) 4-chamber view in ventricular systole of cAVSD. (b) 4-chamber view in ventricular diastole of cAVSD showing single AV valve orifice.

Chapter 13

Abnormal ventriculoarterial connections

Introduction

A normal 4-chamber view of the heart identifies the atria and ventricles and demonstrates normal atrioventricular connections but extended views are necessary to identify the great arteries as they leave the heart thus defining ventriculoarterial connections. Abnormal ventriculoarterial connections that are part of complex lesions are considered with the relevant lesion in other parts of the book.

Transposition of the great arteries

Incidence

- 5% of CHD with male:female ratio of 3:1.

Anatomy

- 'Discordant ventriculoarterial connections':
  - Aorta arises from the morphological right ventricle.
  - Pulmonary artery arises from the morphological left ventricle.

Associated cardiac anomalies

- In isolation is termed simple TGA.
- VSD is present in up to 40% of cases of TGA.
- Coarctation of the aorta.
- Pulmonary stenosis by several possible mechanisms, often with VSD.
- Aortic stenosis is less common.
- Can also be associated with complex CHD.

Haemodynamics and fetal significance

- Higher oxygen saturation in the pulmonary artery than the aorta may well be important in the development of both closure of DA (see later in this topic) and of postnatal persistent elevation of pulmonary vascular resistance.
- The effect of blood supplying the developing brain having mainly come from SVC and not the placenta is a matter for much debate as its metabolic content as well as oxygen saturation is different from a normally connected heart.

U/S features

- 4-chamber view is usually normal:
  - Offsetting may be very subtle
- Extended views demonstrate discordant arterial connections:
  - Left ventricle gives rise to the artery which divides as it passes posteriorly.
  - Right ventricle gives rise to the artery from which the head and neck vessels arise.
- The two great arteries are in parallel with aorta anterior (Fig. 13.1).
- The arterial valves when seen in the same view are in the same plane as opposed to being at right angles in a normally connected heart (Fig. 13.2).
- A normal 3-vessel view cannot be convincingly obtained.
- Doppler may demonstrate an abnormal pattern or velocity through the arterial valves in the presence of additional pathology.

Evolution and prognosis *in utero*

- The lesion is usually well tolerated *in utero*.
- In some fetuses, the arterial duct and atrial septum become restrictive as indicated by:
  - thickened rigid or hypermobile atrial septum
  - absence of clear colour flow signal through foramen ovale
  - constricted DA on imaging
  - bidirectional Doppler signal in DA.

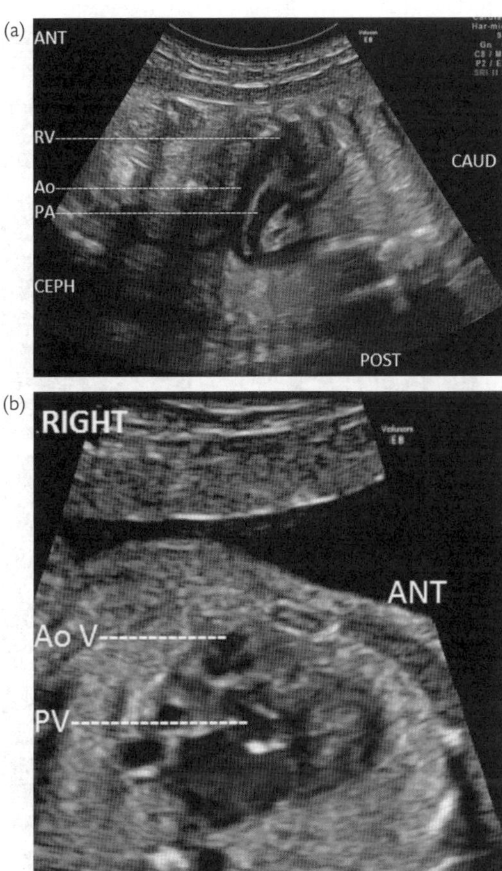

Fig. 13.1 (a) Long-axis view showing great arteries in parallel with Ao anterior arising from RV. (b) Short-axis view showing Ao anterior and to right of PA.

(a)

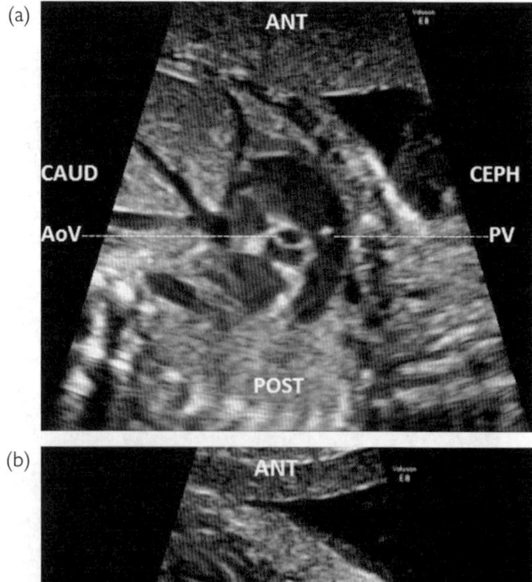

(b)

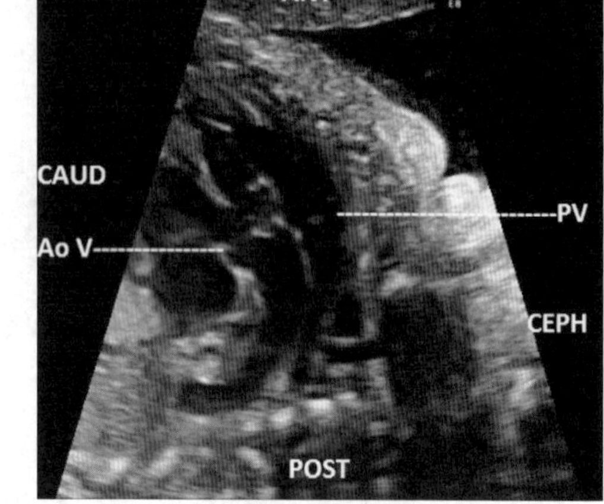

Fig. 13.2 (a) Short-axis view of normally related great arteries in ventricular diastole showing valves in plane at right angles to each other. (b) Long-axis view in TGA in ventricular diastole showing arterial valves in the same plane as each other.

- Monitoring *in utero* is appropriate and evidence of evolving restrictions indicate that early postnatal intervention will be required.
- Absence of echocardiographic evidence of restriction of DA or foramen ovale does not guarantee satisfactory early newborn status.

Association with non-cardiac anomalies

- Simple transposition is usually an isolated lesion having a low association with non-cardiac anomalies.
- TGA is associated with maternal type 1 diabetes:
    - The result of better diabetic monitoring and control is hard to define.
    - The role of gestational or type 2 diabetes is unclear.

Postnatal prognosis and management

- Timing for postnatal intervention will be determined by:
    - size of the foramen ovale
    - presence and size of a VSD
    - size of arterial duct
    - pulmonary vascular resistance.
- Prostaglandin is used to keep the arterial duct patent.
- Balloon atrial septostomy is performed in the early newborn period if mixing of oxygenated and deoxygenated blood is deemed inadequate.
- The arterial switch operation is performed at an interval varying from days to a few weeks.
- Long-term follow-up is appropriate but a normal quality of life is anticipated.

Congenitally corrected transposition of the great arteries

Incidence

- <1% of CHD.

Anatomy

- Normal venoatrial connections.
- Abnormal:
  - atrioventricular connections
  - ventriculoarterial connections.

Haemodynamics

- Double discordancy allows for physiological correction:
  - Blood returning to the heart from the lungs leaves the heart via the aorta, but via the right ventricle.
  - Blood returning from the head, neck, and body leaves the heart through the pulmonary artery, but via the left ventricle.

Associated cardiac conditions

- May be seen in association with:
  - dextrocardia (or mesocardia)
  - VSD in up to 70% (usually perimembranous)
  - pulmonary stenosis (or atresia)
  - aortic stenosis
  - coarctation of the aorta
  - ventricular hypoplasia
  - Ebstein's malformation (or dysplasia) of the systemic (morphological right) atrioventricular valve
  - varying degrees of heart block including complete heart block which may develop *in utero* or postnatally.

U/S features

- Position of the heart might be abnormal.
- Situs solitus or situs inversus.
- Abnormal 4-chamber view (Fig. 13.3):
  - Offsetting reversed.
  - Ventricular spatial relationship often unusual making a good 4-chamber view hard to achieve.
- Great arteries are usually in parallel and in any event with abnormal ventriculoarterial connections.
- Additional anomalies as described previously.
- Bradycardia may be present if heart block occurs.

Evolution and prognosis *in utero*

- Isolated congenitally corrected TGA is usually well tolerated *in utero*.
- Valvar stenosis may progress during pregnancy.
- Systemic AV valve regurgitation may progress but not necessarily until after birth.

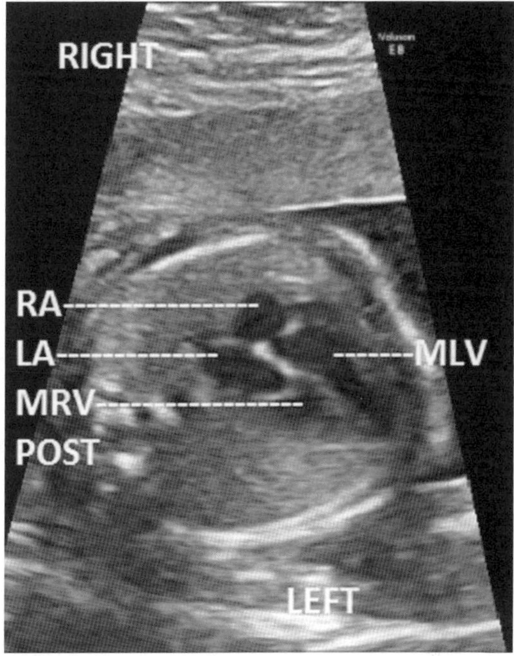

Fig. 13.3 4-chamber view in congenitally corrected TGA showing reversed offsetting of AV valves indicating AV discordance

- Heart rate may slow:
  - 1st- and 2nd-degree heart block progresses to 3rd-degree (complete) heart block.
- Hydrops may develop in severe bradycardia or with severe AV valve regurgitation.

Association with non-cardiac anomalies

- Congenitally corrected TGA is usually an isolated lesion.

Postnatal prognosis and management

- In the absence of other structural cardiac problems or heart block this diagnosis may go unrecognized for decades.
- In time, as a result of the right ventricle serving as the systemic ventricle, signs of right ventricular dysfunction may develop.
- The presence and severity of other cardiac lesions will determine the need for and timing of intervention and define prognosis.

Truncus arteriosus (common arterial trunk)

Incidence

- <1% of CHD.

Anatomy

- Single arterial trunk exits the heart and gives rise to
  - coronary arteries
  - aorta
  - pulmonary arteries.
- In most cases this vessel over-rides a large VSD.
- The 'truncal' valve is usually abnormal:
  - May have 4 leaflets or even more.
  - Usually regurgitant.
  - Can be stenotic.
- Pulmonary arteries arise directly from the arterial trunk but with various different anatomical arrangements:
  - From a single origin from the ascending aorta which soon divides.
  - Adjacent but separate.
  - Separately from opposite sides of the ascending aorta.

Associated cardiac anomalies

- Aortic arch may be right sided.
- Arch may be interrupted.
- Unless arch is interrupted, there is not a DA.

Haemodynamics

- Often well tolerated.
- Truncal valve regurgitation or severe stenosis can cause cardiac failure.

U/S features

- 4-chamber view may be normal.
- 3-vessel view will be abnormal.
- Extended views demonstrate a single vessel leaving the heart overriding the VSD.
- Truncal valve may appear dysplastic on 2D imaging.
- Doppler may demonstrate regurgitation of the truncal valve.
- Pulmonary arteries may be seen arising from the common trunk (Fig. 13.4).
- Interrupted aorta is characterized by a small ascending aorta giving rise to head and neck vessels but no aortic arch.

Prognosis and evolution *in utero*

- Usually well tolerated *in utero*.
- Truncal valve may become progressively regurgitant.

Association with non-cardiac anomalies

- Often (approx. 30%) associated with 22q11 deletion.

Postnatal prognosis and management

- Neonatal surgical repair is usually performed unless other lesions or syndromes contraindicate it.
- Non-cardiac associations have an important impact on survival.

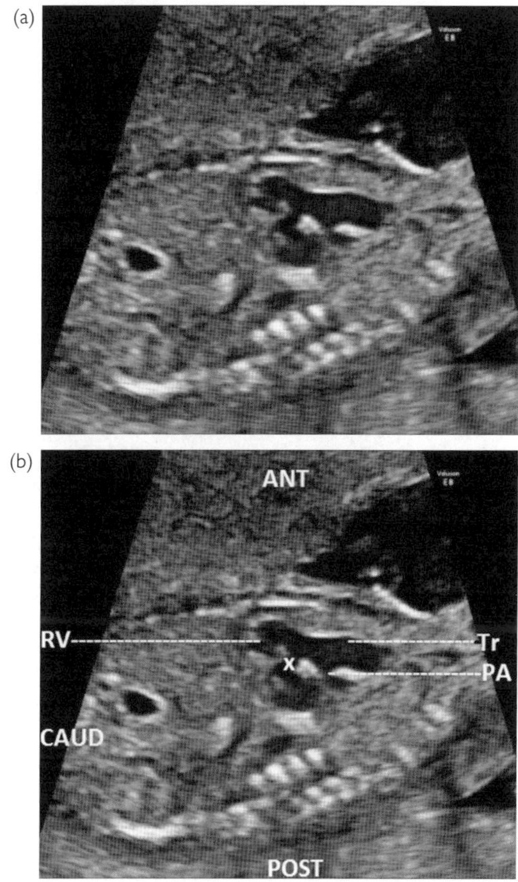

Fig. 13.4 Long axis (a) plain and (b) annotated showing VSD (x) and origin of main PA from arterial trunk.

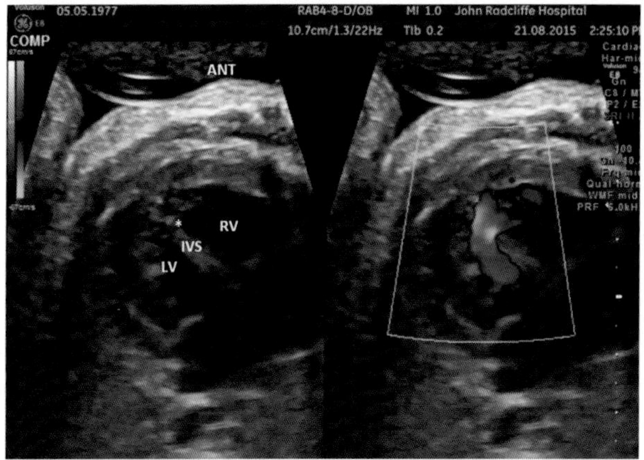

Fig. 6.2 Colour flow Doppler interrogation of interventricular septum (IVS) in 4-chamber view making presence of 1 or more VSDs much clearer than image alone. In colour, signal was blue indicating flow from right (RV) to left ventricle (LV).

(a)

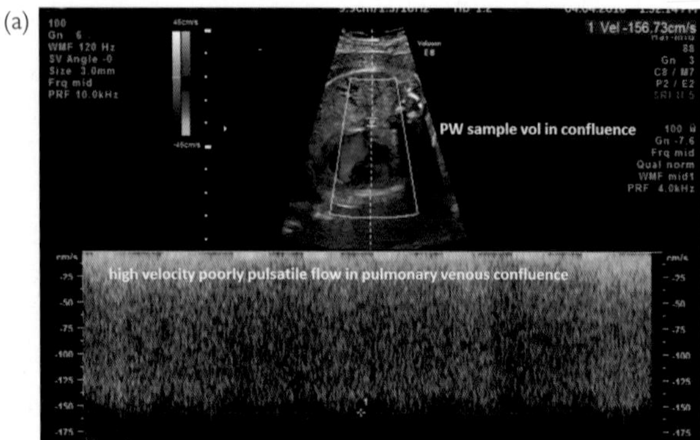

(b)

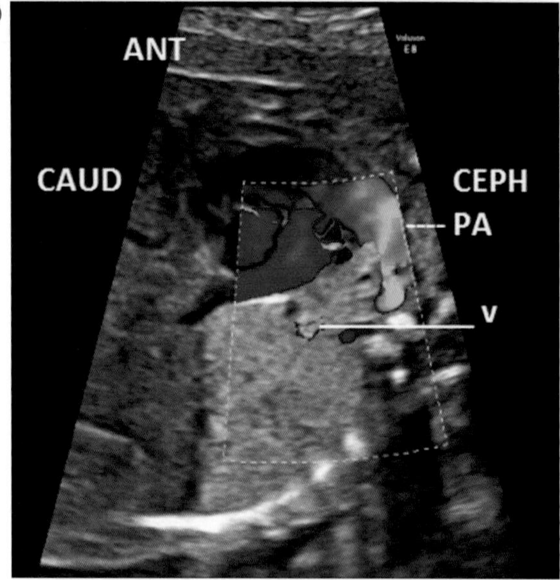

Fig. 10.2 (a) PW Doppler signal in pulmonary venous confluence (v) showing high velocity poorly pulsatile signal indicative of obstruction. (b) Colour flow signal with aliasing in a confluence behind LA.

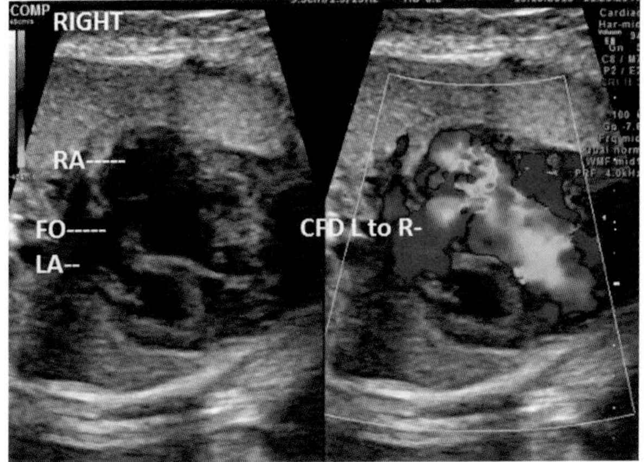

Fig. 10.5 4-chamber view with colour flow Doppler showing L-to-R flow across foramen ovale in left heart obstruction.

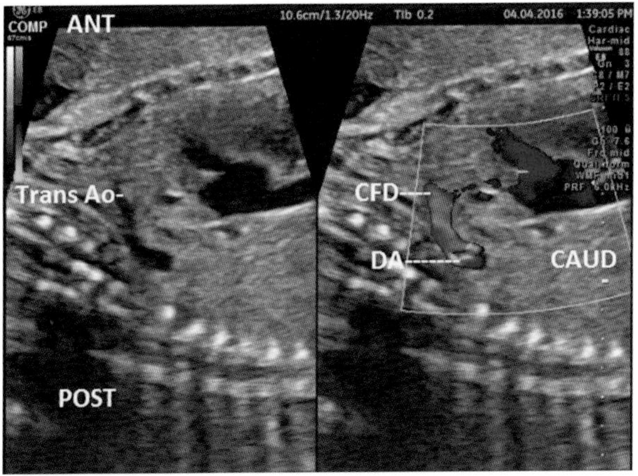

Fig. 10.9 Long-axis view of aortic arch with red colour flow Doppler (CFD) signal indicating flow towards the transducer in the arch, that is to say, retrograde filling from the DA.

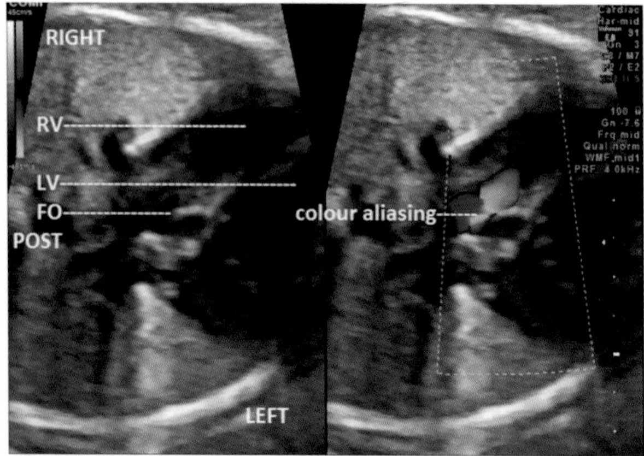

Fig. 10.10 Oblique view of IAS with CFD showing aliasing (i.e. high velocity) in the L-to-R flow across the foramen ovale. Severe left heart obstruction.

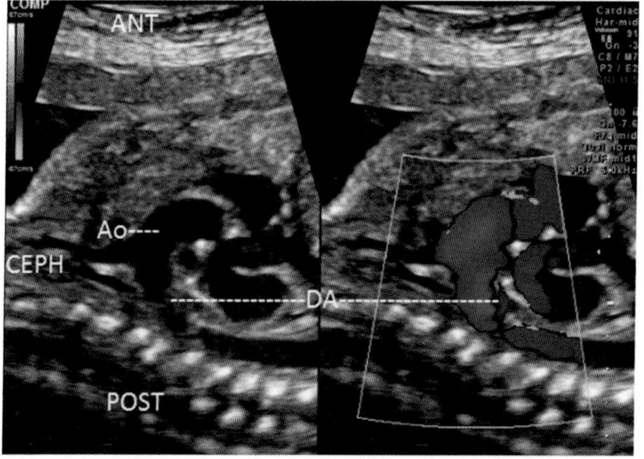

Fig. 11.6 Long-axis view with colour flow Doppler showing retrograde flow in DA in PAIVS.

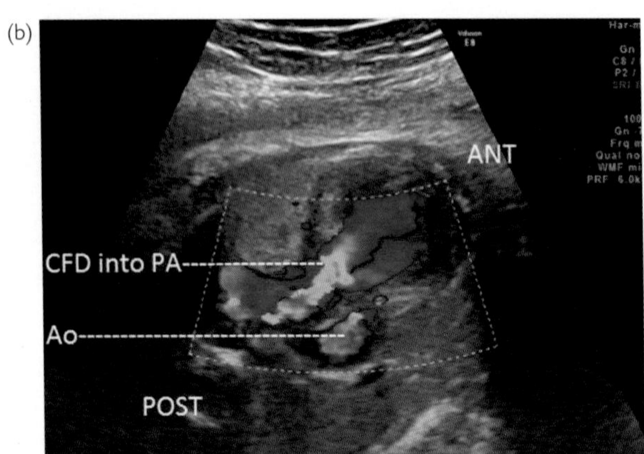

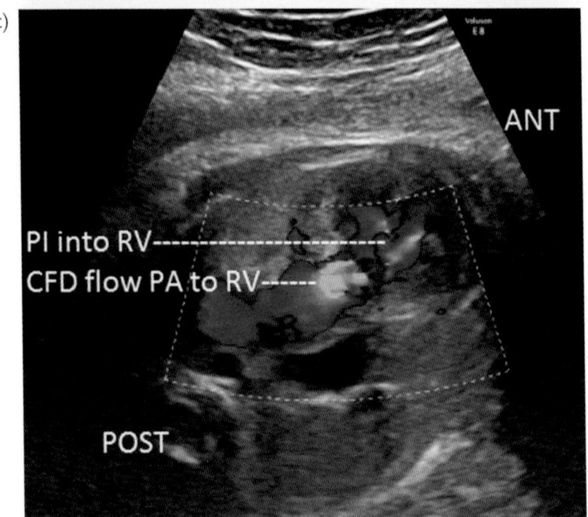

Fig. 11.8 (b) Same view using colour flow Doppler in ventricular systole showing forward flow RV to PA with some acceleration across PV. (c) Same view with colour flow Doppler in ventricular diastole showing PA to RV flow, marked PI in tetralogy of Fallot with APV.

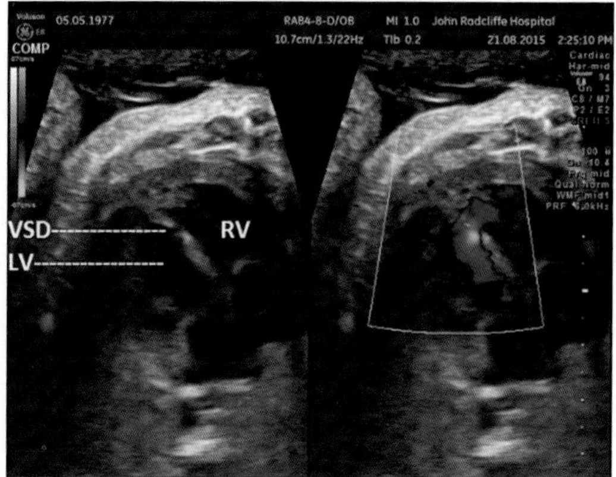

Fig. 12.4 4-chamber view image showing apparently small muscular VSD which with colour flow Doppler is seen to be much larger. The blue Doppler signal reflects flow from RV to LV, the predominant direction in flow for fetal VSD.

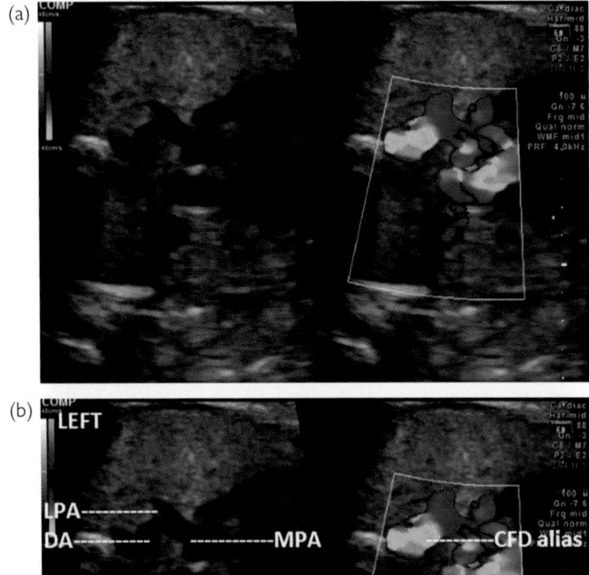

Fig. 24.2 Oblique 3-vessel view showing constriction at the PA end of the DA with increase in blood velocity across that region shown on colour flow Doppler. (a) (plain) and (b) (annotated).

Chapter 14

Miscellaneous abnormalities

Double inlet ventricle

Incidence

- <1% of CHD.

Anatomy

- Both atrioventricular valves open into the same ventricle, virtually always the morphological left ventricle.
- Double inlet right ventricle is exceedingly rare.
- Right ventricle is small and often rudimentary.
- VSD (sometimes termed ventriculobulbar foramen in this context) allows blood entry to rudimentary (usually right) ventricle and the artery arising from it.
- Arterial connections may vary:
  - Normally connected, may have pulmonary outflow obstruction.
  - Transposed, may have systemic outflow obstruction and/or coarctation.

Associated cardiac anomalies

- AV valve stenosis or regurgitation may be present.
- Great arteries may be abnormally related (➲ p. 142).

Haemodynamics

- Right ventricular filling is dependent on the presence of a VSD.
- If VSD is or becomes restrictive, growth of the right ventricle will be further compromised.
- If VSD is restrictive there is in effect obstruction to flow into the artery arising from the rudimentary (right) ventricle.

U/S features

- The 4-chamber view will be abnormal (Fig. 14.1) with the following features:
  - Both inlet valves open into the single ventricle.
  - The small rudimentary ventricle and VSD should be visible.
- Extended views demonstrate arterial disproportion with or without ventriculoarterial discordance (Fig. 14.2).
- Arch views may show a small arch if the risk of duct-dependent coarctation exists.

Evolution and prognosis *in utero*

- This lesion is usually well tolerated during pregnancy.
- VSD may become restrictive.
- Arterial disproportion may increase.

Association with non-cardiac anomalies

- Usually an isolated lesion.

Postnatal prognosis and management

- May be DA dependent.
- Surgical correction is not achievable and treatment is palliative and depends on the anatomical variation but may include:
  - systemic-to-pulmonary arterial shunt if inadequate flow to the lungs

- repair of coarctation with pulmonary artery banding if TGA
- procedure to bypass restrictive VSD in TGA (Damus–Kaye–Stansel operation) or VSD enlargement
- Glenn procedure around 6–12 months of age
- completion of total cavopulmonary connection before school age.

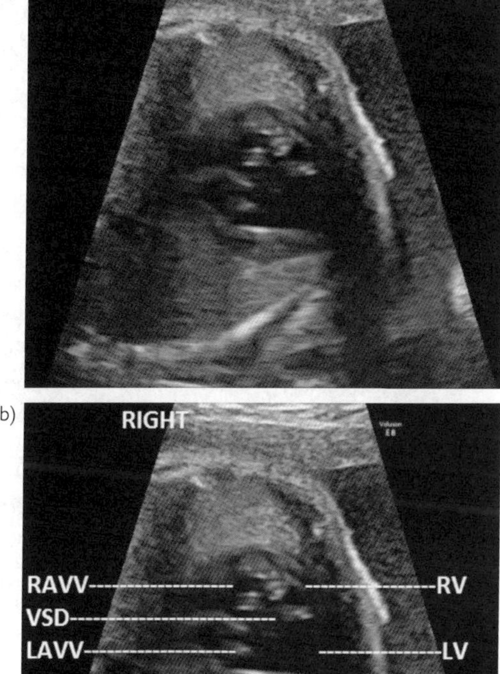

Fig. 14.1 4-chamber view plain (a) and (b) annotated. Both AV valves open predominantly into LV. Small RV accessed through VSD.

(a)

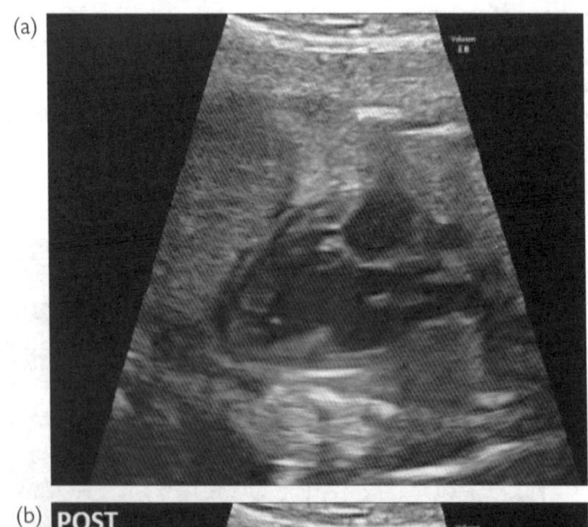

(b)

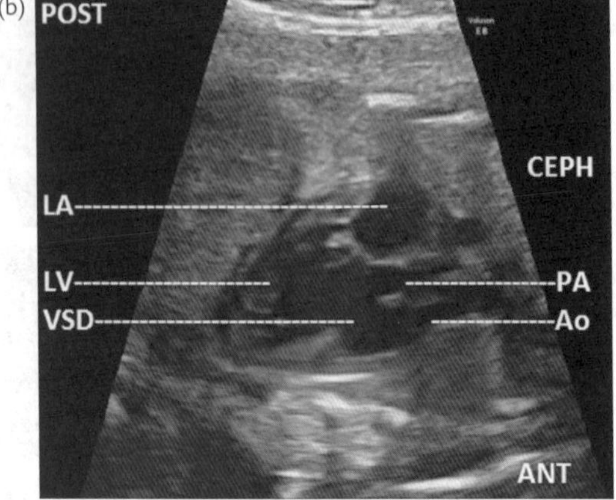

Fig. 14.2 Long-axis view double inlet left ventricle and TGA plain (a) and annotated (b) showing large LV, VSD, small RV and great arteries in parallel with Ao anterior.

Disorders of laterality

The usual arrangement of viscera (morphologic left lung and left atrium on the left, stomach and spleen on the left, liver on the right) is termed situs solitus. The complete mirror image of this is situs inversus. Situs ambiguus is the term traditionally used to describe all other abnormalities of situs although many cases are either bilateral right-sidedness (dextro-isomerism) or left-sidedness (laevo-isomerism). Although some cases have features of both categories, the most typical features of each are described in this topic. See also dextrocardia and heart and stomach on opposite sides ➲ Chapters 15 and 16.

Incidence isomerism (left or right or truly ambiguous)

- Approximately 2% of CHD, 1% of neonates with symptomatic CHD.
- Commoner if parents are consanguineous.

Anatomy (including associated cardiac and non-cardiac anomalies)

Left atrial isomerism

- Bilateral left-sidedness, the classic features include the following:
    - Bilateral left atria.
    - Interruption of IVC which therefore does not drain into right atrium.
    - Azygous (right side) or hemiazygous (left side) venous continuation of the IVC passing through the diaphragm and behind the heart posterior to the descending aorta and entering either a left or right SVC (➲ Fig. 11.1).
    - Hepatic veins drain directly into the atrial mass even in the occasional case in which the IVC is not interrupted.
    - In up to 30% of cases there is either a VSD or complete AVSD.
    - There may be dextrocardia, mesocardia (heart in midline), or a normally positioned heart.
    - Cardiomyopathy may be present or develop through gestation, usually LV non-compaction with varying degrees of myocardial systolic dysfunction.
    - In the absence of a morphological right atrium (site of the sinus node), the rhythm is nevertheless usually AV conduction with normal AV conduction times.
    - Varying degrees of heart block may develop, usually during the 2nd trimester.
    - Complete heart block may be the presenting feature; cardiomyopathy is usually present also in these cases.
- Possible abnormalities of abdominal organs include the following:
    - Presence of multiple spleens.
    - Occasionally biliary atresia (difficult to exclude prenatally).
    - Stomach may be on right.
    - Intestinal rotation is always abnormal although this does not cause volvulus in the majority.
    - Careful planning of multidisciplinary postnatal assessments of these features is important.
- With increasingly accurate screening, more cases of left isomerism without haemodynamically significant cardiac findings are detected. The splenic, intestinal, and hepatic issues still need to be evaluated.

Right atrial isomerism

- There is bilateral right sidedness and asplenia (Ivemark syndrome), features include the following:
  - Bilateral right atria.
  - Aorta and IVC are often both on the same side of the aorta at the level of the diaphragm.
  - Anomalous pulmonary venous drainage (no morphological left atrium) either to innominate vein or SVC/atrial junction.
  - Complete AVSD which may be 'unbalanced' with one ventricle significantly bigger than the other.
  - Double outlet right ventricle with both arteries committed to the RV.
  - Malposition of the great arteries with aorta anterior to the pulmonary artery.
  - Pulmonary stenosis (or atresia).
  - Bilateral SVCs with absent coronary sinus.
  - Cardiac malposition including dextrocardia.
- In addition, abnormalities of abdominal situs are frequently seen in association:
  - Stomach may be midline or on the right side.
  - The same situation exists with respect to risk of volvulus as in left isomerism.
  - Liver is usually midline.
  - Asplenia is usual in this situation (relevant to postnatal prophylactic antibiotic and immunization).
  - Thorough postnatal assessment of these matters is important.

Ultrasound features of isomerism states

- Position of IVC and aorta at diaphragm as described previously.
- Heart and stomach side must be confirmed.
- 4-chamber view may be abnormal.
- Disproportion of ventricles or great arteries common.
- Abnormal rhythm (heart block) may be seen in left isomerism.
- Spongy myocardium in LV may be seen in left isomerism.
- Doppler may reveal regurgitant AV valve(s) or stenosed/atretic pulmonary outflow.

Non-cardiac anomalies

- Most of the non-cardiac structural anomalies associated with this group of cardiac anomalies were mentioned previously.
- Association with chromosome anomalies is rare.

Prognosis

- The more serious cardiac anomalies may be associated with a poor outcome:
  - Duct-dependent circulation is more likely with right atrial isomerism.
  - In some, the cardiac anatomy is such that only palliative surgical procedures are possible.
  - Complete heart block with or without cardiomyopathy may lead to hydrops and has a particularly poor prognosis.
- Asplenia is associated with an increased risk of bacterial sepsis.
- Recurrence risk for this group of cardiac anomalies is probably higher than for other forms of CHD and may be as high as 10%.

Chapter 15

Abnormalities at a glance

Introduction

- Although defining a precise cardiac anomaly can be challenging, it is sometimes immediately obvious that there is something wrong with either the anatomy or rhythm and that further assessment is needed.
- First impressions might suggest abnormalities of:
  - cardiac position
  - heart size
  - chamber disproportion
  - arterial disproportion
  - rhythm disturbance
  - reduced contractility.
- The following tables summarize the most frequently demonstrated deviations from normal and list the differential diagnoses which should be considered in the presence of specific observations.
- Further information on the diagnoses can be found in the relevant chapters.

Abnormal appearances of the cardiac chambers

- The features of a normal 4-chamber view of the heart are described in ➲ Chapter 6 and include:
  - the heart is on the left and occupies ⅓ of the chest
  - RA size is the same as LA
  - RV is slightly larger than LV (especially in 3rd trimester) although both reach the apex.
- See Table 15.1.

Table 15.1 Abnormal appearances of the cardiac chambers

Observation	Consider
Big right atrium	Tricuspid atresia Ebstein's anomaly Tricuspid dysplasia Idiopathic dilated RA, rare Absent ductus venosus, umbilical vein draining directly to RA
Small right atrium	Usually a reflection of enlarged left atrium
Big left atrium	Left AV valve regurgitation Aortic stenosis/atresia
Small left atrium	Hypoplastic left heart syndrome Coarctation of the aorta Total anomalous pulmonary venous drainage
Big right ventricle	Normal variant Coarctation of the aorta Hypoplastic left heart Cardiomyopathy Constriction or premature closure of arterial duct Absent pulmonary valve syndrome RV diverticulum
Small right ventricle	Tricuspid atresia Pulmonary atresia with intact ventricular septum Double inlet left ventricle Unbalanced AVSD
Big left ventricle	Severe aortic stenosis Cardiomyopathy Obstructive right heart lesions

Table 15.1 (*Contd*)

Observation	Consider
Small left ventricle	Normal variant Coarctation of the aorta Hypoplastic left heart Interrupted aortic arch Mitral atresia Aortic atresia Double outlet right ventricle Unbalanced AVSD
Uniformly big heart	Severe intrauterine growth restriction (small chest) Cardiomyopathies Hyperdynamic circulation, including: • anaemia • arteriovenous fistula
Atria bigger than ventricles	Restrictive cardiomyopathy
Uniformly small heart	Non-cardiac anomalies including: • cystadenomatous malformations of the lungs • large pleural effusions • tracheal atresia
Lack of off-setting of the AV valves	cAVSD pAVSD Inlet VSD Other structural anomaly In some fetuses with trisomy 21 and otherwise structurally normal hearts
Exaggerated off-setting	Ebstein's anomaly
Reversed off-setting	Congenitally corrected TGA

Abnormal appearances of the great arteries

- The normal appearance of the great arteries are described in ➲Chapter 6 and include:
  - PA bigger than Ao, in late gestation diameter ratio up to 1.4:1
  - arteries cross as they leave their respective ventricle
  - arterial valves at right angles to each other.
- See Table 15.2.

Table 15.2 Abnormal appearances of the great arteries

Observation	Consider
PA significantly bigger than Ao	PS Coarctation of the aorta Hypoplastic left heart syndrome Aortic stenosis or atresia Absent pulmonary valve
Aorta bigger than pulmonary artery	Pulmonary atresia Tetralogy of Fallot Pulmonary atresia with VSD DORV with subaortic VSD and PS ('Fallot type')
Arteries in parallel without cross-over	Transposition of the great arteries Congenitally corrected TGA DORV with subpulmonary VSD 'TGA-type'
Only 1 artery visible	Pulmonary atresia Aortic atresia Hypoplastic left heart syndrome Common arterial trunk

Abnormalities of cardiac position

- This subject is described in detail in ➔ Chapter 16.
- It is essential to establish left and right sides of the fetus at the beginning of the scan.
- See Table 15.3.

Table 15.3 Abnormalities of cardiac position

Observation	Consider
Heart on right with apex to right	Situs inversus Heterotaxy: • left or right isomerism
Heart on right with apex to left	Mediastinal shift: • space-occupying lesion in left chest or • right lung hypoplasia
Heart midline, apex anywhere	Normal variant Any of the above

Abnormal cardiac axis

The cardiac axis is normally defined as at 45 degrees and to the left of the midline; in the absence of an explanation in terms of an abnormality within the chest or abdomen, significant changes in this angle by $\pm$ 20 degrees, may be a marker for a structural cardiac lesion, particularly:

- tetralogy of Fallot
- pulmonary atresia with VSD.

Abnormalities of the 3VT view

- Criteria for a normal 3-vessel trachea view (3VT) are described in ➲ Chapter 7 and include:
  - PA > Ao > SVC
  - arterial duct and aorta joining as a 'V' to the left of the trachea
  - direction of flow the same in both vessels.
- For many lesions with an abnormal 3VT view, abnormalities in the 4-chamber and great artery views will already have been demonstrated and will feature in the earlier tables in this chapter
- See Table 15.4.

Table 15.4 Abnormal 3VT view

Abnormal observation	Consider
Vessel size	
A. Small aorta	*Forward flow across LVOT* • Coarctation of the aorta *Retrograde flow across LVOT* • Aortic atresia • HLHS *Retrograde flow in transverse or distal Ao* • Severe/critical AS • Interrupted aortic arch
B. Small pulmonary artery/ductal arch	*Forward flow across RVOT* • Tetralogy of Fallot • Ebstein's anomaly • Tricuspid atresia *Retrograde flow across RVOT* • Pulmonary atresia
C. Dilated aorta	*Post-stenotic dilatation of the aortic valve* • Tetralogy of Fallot/PA with VSD
D. Dilated pulmonary artery	*Post stenotic dilatation in PS* • Tetralogy of Fallot with absent pulmonary valve
E. Dilated SVC	*Anaemia* • Cerebral AV malformation • Left atrial isomerism with azygous continuation of IVC to SVC • Supracardiac TAPVD
Vessel alignment	*Abnormal* • TGA • DORV

Table 15.4 (*Contd*)

Abnormal observation	Consider

Vessel number	*2 vessels*
	• Single great artery
	  • Other artery tiny due to atretic valve
	  • Common arterial trunk
	• TGA*
	• DORV*
	* 2 arteries present but only 1 visible on 3VT due to arrangement

	4 vessels • Bilateral SVC (often with prominent coronary sinus into which left SVC drains) • Double aortic arch
Relationship to trachea	*Ao right side of trachea* • Right aortic arch (Ao and PA meet as 'U' behind trachea *Ao seems to be both sides of trachea* • Double aortic arch • Vascular ring *Ao and DA both to right of trachea (meet as a 'V')* • Right duct + right aortic arch
Abnormal Doppler pattern	*Flow in opposite directions* • Atresia or critical stenosis of an arterial valve • Retrograde filling of that artery via duct *Unexpected additional signals (on colour flow Doppler)* • Aberrant vessels

Abnormal cardiac rhythms

- Features of a normal cardiac rhythm are described in ➔ Chapter 16 (cardiac rhythm) and include:
  - regular rhythm at rate 120–160 bpm
  - transient episodes of sinus bradycardia, especially in the 2nd trimester.
- Irregular heart rate is usually due to atrial ectopic beats which are common, usually benign, and a normal variant. See Table 15.5.

Table 15.5 Abnormalities of cardiac rhythm

Observation	Consider
Tachycardia (>160 bpm)	Sinus tachycardia (rarely >180 bpm) SVT, including atrial flutter (usually >200 bpm) Ventricular tachycardia (very rare in the fetus)
Bradycardia (<110 bpm)	Sinus bradycardia (many causes) Blocked atrial ectopic beats 2nd- or 3rd-degree heart block
Irregular heart rate (usually with periods of normal heart rate)	Atrial ectopic beats, blocked and/or conducted See ➔ Chapter 16 for rarer causes

Chapter 16

Abnormal cardiac position

Normal cardiac position and axis

Situs solitus

- This is the normal arrangement; the heart:
  - lies in the left side of the chest—laevocardia
  - apex points to the left at an angle of 45 degrees (normal range 30–60 degrees) as measured by the angle of the ventricular septum and a perpendicular anteroposterior line through the spine.
- The IVC is to the right of the spine and anterior to the aorta on the left side of the spine.
- The stomach is in the left side of the abdomen.

To confirm these relationships, it is important to get a 4-chamber view in a true cross-section of the chest with a complete rib on each side; an oblique view may give a false impression of heart size and position.

Most structurally and functionally abnormal hearts have situs solitus, but this can never be assumed

Abnormalities of cardiac position

Alterations in the position of the heart may be due to:

- cardiac abnormality or
- non-cardiac intrathoracic structural anomaly.

Structural cardiac anomalies

- Lesions recognized to be associated with an abnormal position, especially in early gestation, include:
  - tetralogy of Fallot (increased angle)
  - double outlet right ventricle
  - pulmonary atresia with VSD
  - congenitally corrected TGA (dextrocardia in about 50%).
- Situs solitus with heart and apex to the right (sometimes called dextroposition):
  - Very rare.
  - Apex points downwards or to the right.
  - Other features of situs solitus (➔ p. 174).
  - Absence of other thoracic pathology.
  - Associated with structural heart abnormalities, may be minor.
  - May be distinguishable from dextrocardia due to pulmonary abnormality when the apex usually points to the left.
- Situs inversus—a rare condition in which there is a mirror image arrangement of thoracic and abdominal organs:
  - Heart (and apex) is to the right side in the chest (dextrocardia).
  - Stomach on the right in abdomen.
  - Right aortic arch.
  - Descending aorta is right of spine at the diaphragm.
  - Liver mainly on left.
  - Spleen on the right.
  - IVC is on the left of the spine.
  - The heart is usually normal although any structural abnormality may be present including congenitally corrected TGA.
  - There may be other family members with similar anatomy.
  - Genetics are complex.
  - A proportion may be associated with cilial dysmotility.
- Heterotaxy/isomerism states:
  - The heart may be on the right or the left with apex pointing to the same side.
  - there are often significant cardiac abnormalities (➔ Chapter 14).
  - An essentially normal heart can occur, more commonly in left isomerism.
  - Stomach position varies or may be midline.
  - Systemic or pulmonary venous drainage is usually abnormal depending on whether there is left or right isomerism.
- Ectopia cordis:
  - The heart is partly or completely outside the thoracic cavity.
  - There is usually an abnormal cardiac structure.
  - In particular, double outlet right ventricle.
  - May be part of the syndrome of pentalogy of Cantrell, including omphalocele, anterior diaphragmatic hernia, pericardial defect, sternal cleft.

Abnormality of development of thoracic contents

- These may have secondary effects on the position and/or orientation of the heart.
- Disorders include:
  - congenital diaphragmatic hernia (Fig. 16.1), associated with increased risk of CHD
  - cystadenomatous malformation of the lung
  - other rarer lung tumours
  - compression due to pleural and/or pericardial fluid
  - unilateral pulmonary hypoplasia/aplasia, including sequestration and abnormal venous as in Scimitar syndrome.
- In all these situations the apex usually still points to the left.
- Occasionally the primary abnormality is of abdominal contents, particularly large exomphalos.

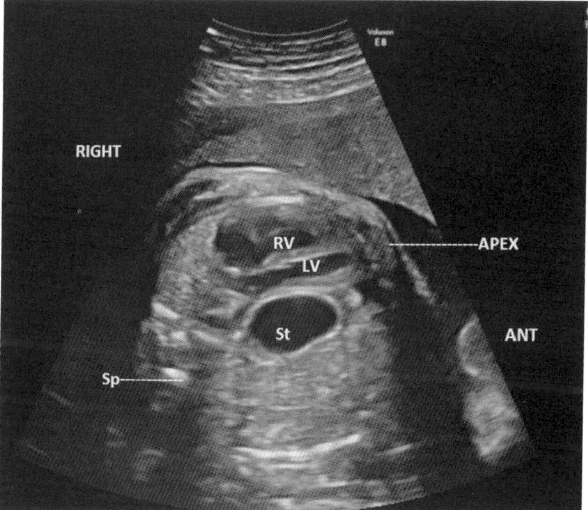

Fig. 16.1 Cross-section through chest, well orientated (symmetrical ribs seen on both sides of thorax) showing heart and apex displaced rightward due to a large left congenital diaphragmatic hernia with stomach in the chest in the same transverse plane as the heart.

Chapter 17

Fetal cardiac rhythm

Introduction

Normal cardiac rhythm originates in the sinus node, a right atrial structure. Atrial electrical depolarization is manifest on the ECG by a P wave and is followed by atrial contraction.

Conduction to the ventricle is through the atrioventricular node and the bundle of His (Fig. 17.1). Ventricular depolarization produces the QRS complex on the ECG and is followed by ventricular contraction.

The interval between atrial and ventricular depolarization is measured as the PR interval on a surface ECG. In the fetus, it is the consequence of depolarization that is detected—either muscle contraction or blood flow. In sinus rhythm every atrial contraction is initiated from the sinus node and is followed by a ventricular one and every ventricular contraction is preceded by an atrial one originating from the sinus node. The interval between atrial and ventricular activity in the fetus is 110–140 msec, depending on the method used, gestation (interval increases with advancing gestation), and resting heart rate. Serial measurements using the same method by the same observer are desirable if sequential change is being looked for (as in maternal antibody cases).

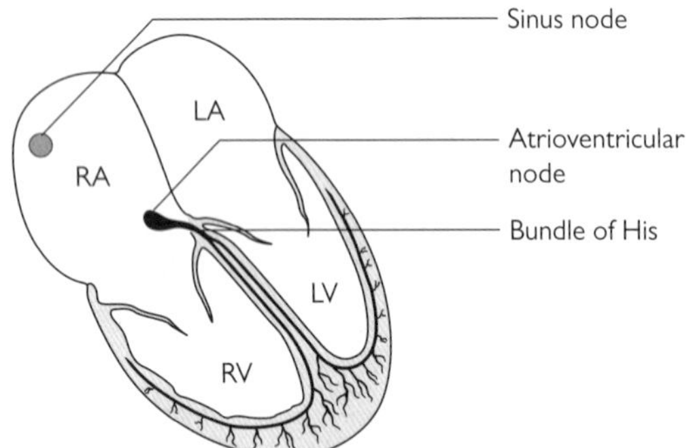

Fig. 17.1 Normal conduction pathways. Electrical activity can only pass from atrial mass to ventricular tissue via the AV node and bundle of His.

Identification of cardiac rhythm

Fetal ECG technology currently cannot be used as a standard clinical tool to diagnose cardiac rhythm. There are several ways to assess rhythm using ultrasound (Table 17.1):

- M-mode echocardiography, by placing the cursor through an atrial wall and a ventricular wall simultaneously (Fig. 17.2).
- Doppler echocardiography, using PW with a large enough sample volume to interrogate simultaneously either:
  - LV inflow and outflow or
  - SVC and ascending aorta or
  - pulmonary artery and vein (Fig. 17.3) which is easier than Ao/SVC.
- Tissue Doppler imaging has been used to evaluate fetal AV conduction times but is not in widespread clinical use.

Table 17.1 Relative advantages of ways of echocardiographic assessment of fetal heart rhythm and AV time

	M-mode	PW LV in/out	PW A Ao/SVC	PW PA/PV
Ease	++	++	+	+++
Rhythm	++	++	+++	+++
AV time	+	++	+++	+++

Each + indicates relative strength of technique.
A Ao, ascending aorta; AV, atrioventricular; LV, left ventricle/ventricular; PA, pulmonary artery; PV, pulmonary vein; PW: pulsed wave; SVC: superior vena cava.

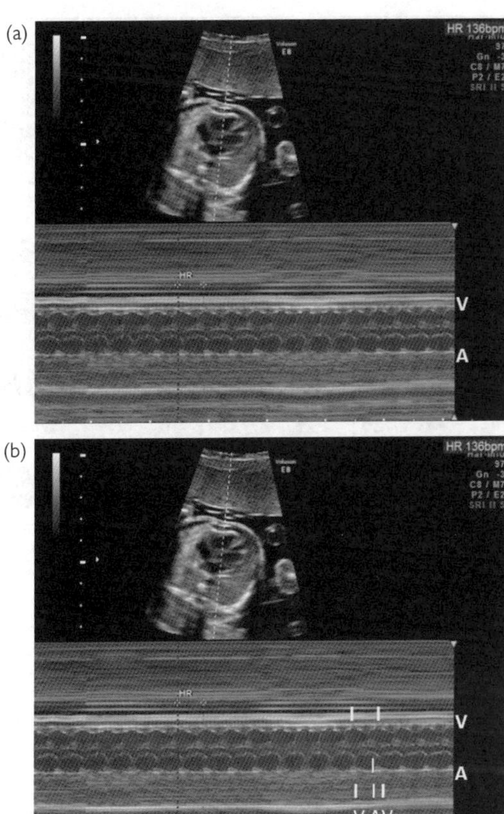

Fig. 17.2 (a) M-mode of SR showing atrial (A) and ventricular (V) contractions and calculation of heart rate (136/min) by measuring the time between the same part of the cardiac cycle in 2 consecutive cycles. (b) The same M-mode trace showing the onset of ventricular (**I**) and atrial (I) contractions and how VA and VA intervals can be identified. In this case the rhythm is a long VA one, a feature of SR as well as of some less common forms of SVT.

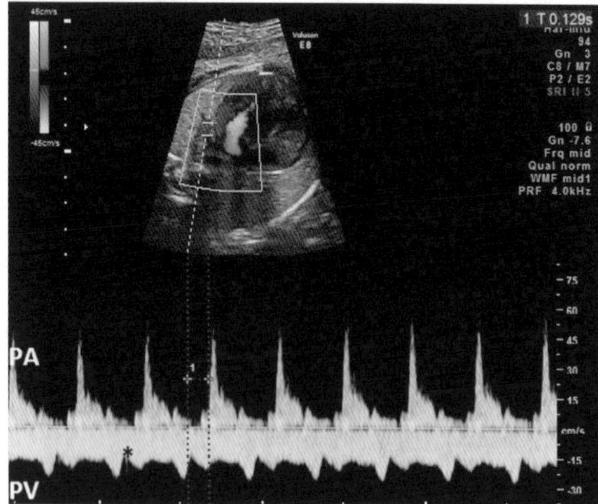

Fig. 17.3 PW Doppler waveforms from PA and PV, showing the 'dip' in velocity in pulmonary vein (pv) which signifies atrial systole (*) and the arterial waveform in ventricular systole allowing accurate measurement of the AV conduction time, in this case 129 msec (normal).

Normal rhythms

Sinus rhythm (SR)

Fetal heart rate can reach 180/min up to 10 weeks' gestation and falls to between 110 and 160 by 12–14 weeks. After 14 weeks, rates outside this range warrant careful assessment of rhythm as they may indicate pathology.

Sudden transient sinus bradycardia

Can be physiological if it has the following features:
- Occurs before 32 weeks, much less common thereafter.
- Occurs only infrequently, not more than twice in 10 minutes.
- Bradycardia lasts not more than 10–15 beats.
- Return to normal is by gradual increase in rate over 5–10 seconds.
- Parameters of fetal well-being are normal.
- Basic cardiac rhythm is sinus.
- Heart function is normal.
- No evidence of onset of labour.

Sustained sinus bradycardia (<110/min)

- Rarely normal even if no haemodynamic compromise.
- See ➲ p. 200 for detailed consideration.

Sinus tachycardia (consistently >160/min)

Requires evaluation:
- Confirmation of rhythm by echocardiography (Figs 17.2 and 17.3):
  - 1:1 AV conduction.
  - Atrial activity precedes ventricular by normal interval with VA longer than AV (➲ p. 183).
  - Rate rarely sustained above 180/min.
  - Rate varies with fetal activity and sleep state.
- Full assessment of fetal well-being.
- Exclude:
  - Labour.
  - Fetal sepsis.
- Consider maternal causes:
  - Pyrexia, any cause.
  - Thyrotoxicosis, active or previously treated.
  - Drugs/medication, e.g. sympathomimetics, excessive caffeine intake.
- Does not require treatment in and of itself.

Atrial (supraventricular) ectopics

Atrial ectopics/supraventricular ectopics (SVEs) are a common normal variant which usually resolve within a few weeks of detection. They are also termed premature atrial contractions (PACs). They can either be:
- conducted to the ventricle or
- not conducted (blocked).

They are frequently first detected as an irregular heart beat during routine midwifery evaluation.

Diagnosis of SVEs

- Can often be strongly suspected without echocardiographic assessment of rhythm if heart rate by Doppler or cardiotocograph (CTG) shows the following features:
  - Is essentially regular with either occasional pause (if SVE blocked) or apparent early beat followed by a pause (if SVE conducted).
  - Suddenly slows by a recognizable fraction of the normal sinus rate and suddenly reverts back or changes to a different slow and/or irregular rate. The pattern depends on SVE frequency, regularity in relation to sinus beats and whether blocked or conducted. Thus heart rates will be 65–90 and regular if SVEs alternate with sinus beats (that is 1:1) and somewhat faster but irregular if 1:2 or 1:3 relationship SVE to sinus beat occurs.
  - Runs of several minutes of 1:1 sinus:blocked ectopic producing slow and regular heart rhythm are quite common.
- Any of the echocardiographic methods for determining fetal rhythm can be used for precise diagnosis (Fig. 17.4).

Significance of SVEs

SVEs are common and normal, and usually of no significance but:

- can cause anxiety to family and professionals
- rarely occur in labour but if frequent can make monitoring difficult
- blocked SVEs if not recognized as such can result in unnecessary intervention for fetal bradycardia
- SVEs are associated with an increased risk of fetal (and neonatal) supraventricular tachycardia (SVT):
  - this is because at any age SVT can be initiated by an atrial ectopic in susceptible individuals
  - the risk of SVT appears to be greater if ectopics are blocked.
  - overall risk of SVT is <5%.
- SVEs are more frequent if the fossa ovalis balloons from right to left atrium toward the mitral valve (Fig. 17.5). This rarely has any other significance to the fetus and often resolves after birth.

Management of SVEs

- Referral for detailed cardiac assessment is not required if:
  - fetal health normal
  - labour not commenced
  - criteria/features given previously apply
  - resolve over timescale of a few weeks
  - local protocol for irregular fetal heart known in antenatal clinics (see Box 17.1).
- Detailed cardiac assessment involves:
  - rhythm diagnosis
  - definition of heart structure and function
  - plan for follow-up.
- If frequent in labour, monitoring is possible with the help of detailed fetal echocardiography but caesarean section becomes more likely.

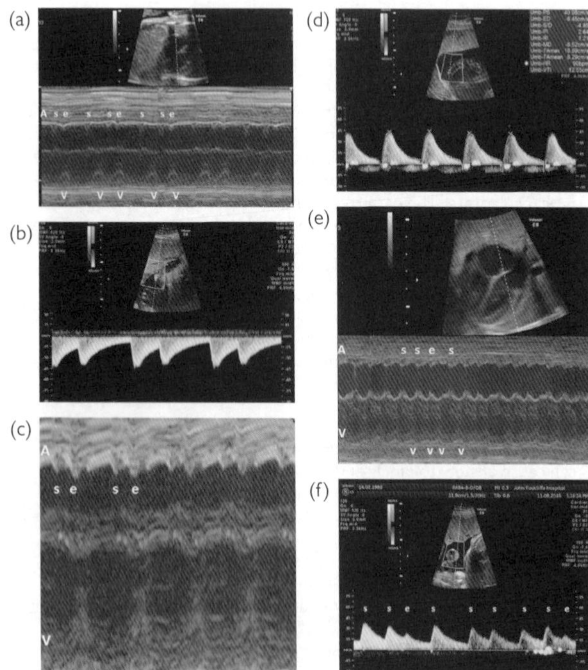

Fig. 17.4 (a) M-mode through atria (A) and ventricles (V). Some atrial contractions are sinus in origin (s) and some are ectopics (e) in a ratio of 2:1. The ectopics are not conducted to V, they are 'blocked'. (b) The same rhythm sequence as manifest by arterial PW signals from the umbilical artery giving an irregular heart rhythm. (c) Enlarged M-mode showing atria (A) and ventricular (V) walls with sinus (s) and ectopic atrial beats (e) alternating. The ectopics are blocked so that ventricular rate is slow (90/min) but regular. (d) umbilical artery Doppler signal in the same case as in (c) showing slow regular arterial pulsations. Blocked atrial ectopics alternating 1:1 with sinus beats. (e) M-mode showing sinus beats (s) and a conducted atrial ectopic (e) all of which result in ventricular contraction (v). The compensatory pause after the conducted e gives an irregular heart rhythm at a normal rate. (f) Umbilical artery Doppler signal showing arterial pulsation after some conducted atrial ectopics and after 3rd from left is a non-conducted one.

- Follow-up:
  - By fetal heart rate assessment every 4–7 days to rule out frequent or sustained SVT until SVEs resolve, this can be done by referring midwifery service.
  - If resolve before term, no neonatal assessment required.
  - If present at term or in labour, arrange neonatal ECG for rhythm and for pre-excitation (indicates an additional increased risk for SVT).
  - If SVT noted, irrespective of duration, follow SVT assessment and treatment protocol as discussed on ➔ p. 190.

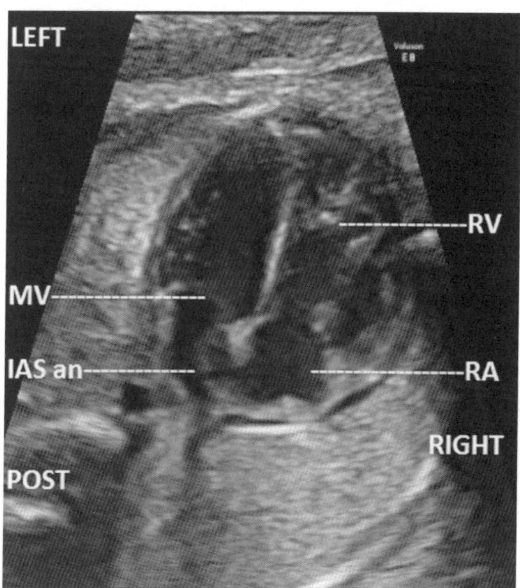

Fig. 17.5 4-chamber view in ventricular systole showing aneurysm (an) of IAS bowing from RA towards MV in left atrium.

Box 17.1 Irregular fetal heart rate detected at a midwifery check

If other parameters of fetal health are normal, this is likely to be due to atrial ectopics

Urgent referral to fetal cardiology is indicated at any stage the heart rate is:

- sustained, regular and slow (<110) or
- fast (>180).

Otherwise follow 1–4 below:

1. If infrequent ectopics, reassure and arrange to listen again in 1 week.
2. If persist at 1 week, refer to hospital antenatal department for confirmation of findings.
3. If antenatal department confirm findings, observe weekly for another 2 weeks.
4. If still present then refer to fetal cardiology.

Fast abnormal rhythms

These present from 16 weeks' gestation onwards with:
- heart rate above 160 bpm or
- fetal hydrops.

They can be either:
- supraventricular or
- ventricular.

General evaluation of fetal tachycardia

History
- Parental or other family history of relevance:
  - arrhythmias
  - cardiomyopathy
- Maternal drug ingestion (sympathomimetics, excessive caffeine).
- Maternal disease (thyrotoxicosis, current or previous).

Clinical assessment

This involves ascertaining the following:
- Fetal well-being.
- Presence of oedema, pericardial, pleural, or ascitic fluid.
- Heart structure and function:
  - Cardiomyopathy can be primary but more often secondary to arrhythmia.
  - Function should be reassessed when sinus rhythm is established.
- Rate:
  - Usually above 180/min, most often over 200.
  - Incessant or paroxysmal.
  - Percentage of a timed study (15 or 20 minutes) spent in tachycardia.
  - Regular or irregular.
- Identifying cardiac rhythm as precisely as possible (➔ p. 182)
- Noting presence and type of ectopics if periods of sinus rhythm occur.

Sinus tachycardia

This is a normal rhythm and is considered in detail on ➔ p. 186.

Supraventricular tachycardia (SVT)

More than 98% of fetal tachycardias are some form of SVT.

The term fetal SVT includes a variety of different rhythms with atrial flutter being the only one that 2D scanning can identify separately. Thus many publications describe SVT and atrial flutter but do not further classify type of SVT.

Recognition of other types of SVT with M-mode or Doppler echocardiography is often possible and is outlined later in this topic. This clarification may influence management.

Types of SVT

The following tachycardias are classified as supraventricular (Fig. 17.6):

Atrioventricular re-entry tachycardia (AVRT)
- Commonest type of SVT in fetus (60–75%).
- May be sustained or intermittent.

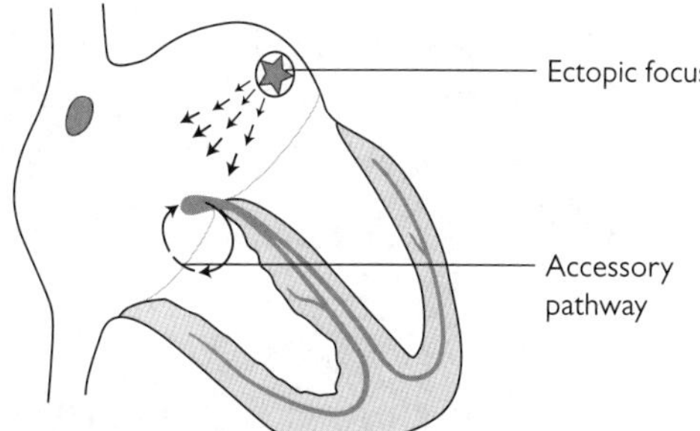

Fig. 17.6 Diagrammatic representation of an AV accessory pathway, the substrate for AVRT, the commonest form of fetal SVT, and of an ectopic focus which could produce atrial ectopic beats or much more rarely an ectopic atrial tachycardia.

- Rate 190–260/min, usually 220–240/min
- Rate varies little in short term.
- Due to an accessory pathway between atria and ventricles
- Occasionally associated with cardiac abnormality especially:
  - Ebstein's malformation of tricuspid valve
  - congenitally corrected transposition
  - cardiac tumours (➔ pp. 220–1).
- Myocarditis/cardiomyopathy.
- On M-mode/Doppler, atrial signal follows ventricular by a shorter time than that to the next ventricular one, short VA time (Fig. 17.7a) equivalent to the RP interval on postnatal ECG.
- In the short term, recurrent episodes are common.
- Most accessory pathways become non-functioning in time, thus predisposition to SVT resolves, sometimes by birth and frequently by 1 year of age.
- Some accessory pathways will be manifest by a pre-excited ECG in sinus rhythm after birth (Wolff–Parkinson–White syndrome).

Atrial flutter (20–25% of fetal SVT)

- Due to a derangement of atrial activity resulting in a circular passage of electrical activity around part of the atrial mass (sometimes termed macro re-entry) producing rapid atrial contractions.
- Atrial rate 350–500/min. (Fig. 17.7b).
- Ventricular rate depends on degree of atrioventricular block but 1:2 is commonest giving rate of 180 to 250/min.
- Degree of block may vary spontaneously or in response to treatment, giving differing ventricular rates and irregularity at times.
- Occasional associations:
  - Accessory pathways.
  - Structural CHD (AVSD in 3–4%).
  - Heart muscle disease, which may be familial.
- Once sinus rhythm restored, recurrences are rare.

(a)

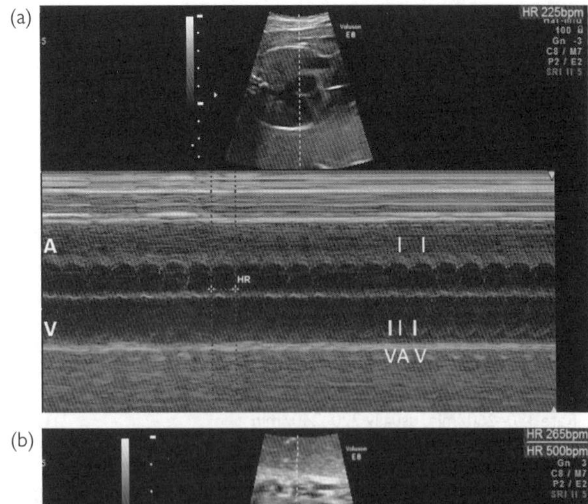

(b)

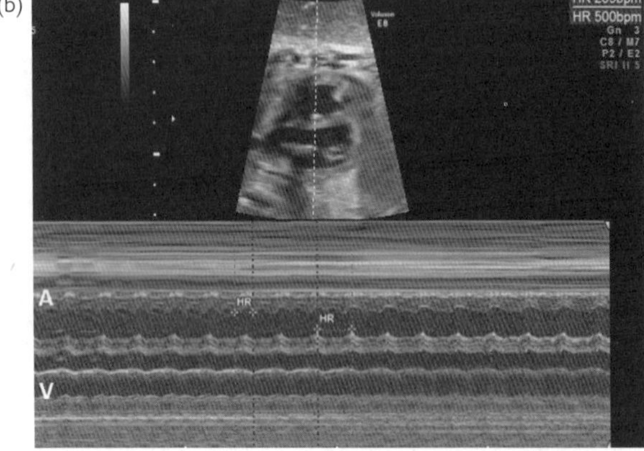

Fig. 17.7 (a) M-mode of SVT (225/min). Onset of atrial (A) and ventricular (V) contractions shown by I and **I** respectively, demonstrating VA time shorter than AV interval. Short VA SVT. (b) M-mode atrial flutter showing atrial rate twice that of ventricular rate. Automatic calculation by machine rarely precisely 2:1 but clearly A:V conduction is 2:1 giving ventricular rate 265/min.

Long VA tachycardias (10–20%)

So named because the interval between ventricular and subsequent atrial contraction is longer than from atrial to next ventricular contraction (ratio VA:AV >1). This is also a feature of SR which can therefore make sinus tachycardia difficult to distinguish (see Fig. 17.2).

Two arrhythmias are characterized by long VA:

- Atrial ectopic tachycardia (AET).
- Permanent junctional reciprocating tachycardia (PJRT).

These cannot be differentiated in the fetus. Both are:

- less likely to be intermittent than AVRT
- likely to be slower than AVRT (sometimes <200/min)
- less likely to respond to digoxin than AVRT or atrial flutter (see Box 17.2)
- less likely than AVRT to resolve in infancy.

Very rare types of fetal SVT

- Junctional ectopic tachycardia (JET):
  - Also called His bundle tachycardia.
  - Slightly irregular ventricular rate.
  - Ventricular rate faster than atrial rate.
  - Treatment as for AVRT but likely to progress to 2nd- or 3rd-line drugs.
- Atrioventricular nodal re-entry tachycardia (AVNRT):
  - Accessory pathway is within AV node.
  - Probably not distinguishable from other forms of SVT on fetal echocardiography (would most commonly have very short VA interval).
  - Treatment would be as for AVRT.
- Multifocal atrial ectopic tachycardia:
  - Also termed chaotic atrial rhythm.
  - AV synchrony varies from beat to beat.
  - Rhythm is fast and irregular.
  - Heart is usually structurally normal.
  - Insufficient evidence to have clear guidelines for fetal therapy but postnatal treatment often initially merely increases AV block and slows ventricular rate rather than restores SR.
  - Treatment with digoxin and/or flecainide seems reasonable.
  - May be associated with Costello syndrome.
  - May be secondary to cardiomyopathy.
  - May resolve in early childhood.

Treatment of SVT

General principles include the following:

- Avoid delivery if possible until SR is restored.
- Observe precautions in list below to avoid cardiac risk to mother receiving antiarrhythmic drugs (see Boxes 17.2 and 17.3).
- Clarify that there is no maternal history:
  - suggestive of arrhythmia or heart muscle disease
  - of concomitant incompatible drug treatment.
- Clarify no paternal or other family history suggestive or serious possibly inheritable cardiac disease.

Box 17.2 Digoxin oral

Check precautions (see 'General principles' list).

Do not use if mother has hypokalaemia or a short PR interval.

- Load 500 micrograms then 250 micrograms 8-hourly.
- Check fetus every 48–72 hours until regimen stable.
- Omit one dose and reduce to 12-hourly if symptoms of toxicity (advise mother about nausea, vomiting, visual disturbance) at any stage.
- After 5 days:
    - check maternal digoxin level (aim to keep in high therapeutic range 6 hours after a dose)
    - repeat maternal ECG.
- Reduce dose as above if:
    - blood level above therapeutic range at 5 days
    - ECG shows changes other than ST/T effects and longer PR interval.
- Carefully review compliance before increasing dose if level low or no ECG changes.
- After 10–14 days:
    - repeat blood potassium, calcium, and drug levels
    - repeat ECG
    - consider altering therapy if no response or if hydrops develops at any stage.
- If fetus in SR at 10–14 days:
    - check fetus weekly
    - maintain dose for at least 4 weeks of SR or until delivery.

- Before administering any drug perform maternal ECG, looking for:
    - conduction disturbance
    - pre-excitation (short PR interval and delta wave)—contraindicates digoxin
    - QRS duration—if prolonged, flecainide would be contraindicated
    - QT interval—if prolonged, amiodarone and flecainide contraindicated
- Before maternal flecainide or any 2nd- or 3rd-line drug treatment is given, obtain a maternal echocardiogram to rule out heart muscle disease.
- Plasma potassium and calcium (abnormalities predispose to maternal adverse effects from drug therapy).
- Start treatment if:
    - >50% of time in SVT
    - cardiac function depressed in SR even if time in SVT <50% (function hard to assess in SVT)
    - SVT <50% of time but detailed frequent follow-up not possible—many will progress to sustained tachycardia and even hydrops
    - any evidence of hydrops (fluid in 2 or more body cavities and/or oedema). A small stable pericardial effusion is acceptable.

Box 17.3 Flecainide oral

Check precautions (see 'General principles' list).

Do not use if maternal ECG has QRS duration above 100 msec or a long QT interval.

- Start at 100 mg 8-hourly.
- Reduce digoxin by one dose a day (flecainide displaces bound digoxin thereby raising blood concentration).
- Assess fetus every 24–48 hours.
- After 24–48 hours, repeat ECG—a slight prolongation of QRS duration is likely.
- Instruct mother to stop drug if she experiences palpitations.
- If drug tolerated, at 5 days:
  - repeat maternal ECG for QRS duration and QTc
  - measure digoxin level if appropriate
  - assess fetus.
- If still in tachyarrhythmia and:
  - maternal QRS duration remains <150 msec with QTc <0.5
  - no fetal or maternal proarrhythmia
  - drug level not toxic.
- Continue 100 mg 8-hourly.
- Cotinine surveillance as above at 3–5-day intervals.
- It may take several weeks to establish SR.
- If SR restored, consider reduction of flecainide to 100 mg 12-hourly.
- If no response/unacceptable side effects/fetus deteriorates, change regimen (➔ p. 196).

- Have protocol for:
  - which drug
  - what dose
  - how/when to monitor mother and fetus.
- Drug therapy:
  - Transplacental, administered to mother by oral or parenteral route.
  - Direct fetal: umbilical vein is preferred, other fetal routes have been used including intramuscular and intra-amniotic.
- Oral maternal therapy is generally preferable and is nearly always appropriate unless:
  - maternal gastrointestinal function seriously impaired
  - deemed necessary to get high fetal blood drug levels quickly
  - adenosine to terminate arrhythmia acutely is indicated (must be into umbilical vein)
  - invasive fetal procedure/sampling indicated for another reason.
- Practice varies but outpatient management is safe if:
  - maternal compliance with medication and understanding of indications and ability to seek advice are good
  - frequent and regular assessment in the clinic is possible for mother
  - a regimen no more complex than oral digoxin and/or flecainide is effective and problem free.

- There are many reported drug regimens for fetal SVT.
- It is important to have a local protocol with a cardiology service taking responsibility for mother and fetus.
- Flecainide is increasingly replacing digoxin as 1st-line treatment although digoxin remains widely used.
- If hydrops develops while on digoxin, then flecainide can be added or substituted in all types except atrial flutter.
- We recommend not using flecainide alone in atrial flutter because of the theoretical, and occasionally observed, risk of producing a faster ventricular rate as the atrial rate slows allowing the degree of AV block to be less. Digoxin protects against this.
- Maternal admission to a cardiology ward is appropriate if:
  - parenteral drug administration is required
  - regimens more complex than digoxin and/or flecainide are used
  - maternal cardiac disease of any kind is present
  - there is any suggestion of maternal arrhythmia while on treatment.

Fetal antiarrhythmic drug doses

If digoxin and flecainide do not work and delivery is deemed unwise, alternative regimens to consider include:

- adenosine into the umbilical vein can be effective but if SR is restored it is likely to be only temporary.
- the longer-term choice is between amiodarone and sotalol used either alone or with digoxin. Amiodarone should only be used if pre-treatment maternal ECG has normal QTc and it does not increase beyond 0.5 on treatment. Acceptable maternal ECG changes on sotalol should be discussed with an adult cardiologist.
- *Standard regimens are not widely agreed for these drugs and must be supervised by a cardiologist.*

Prognosis of SVT

- Untreated, cases of SVT can remain well for weeks but progression to hydrops and death is not rare and cannot be predicted from type of SVT or heart rate.
- Treatment restores SR in 80% or more if not hydropic.
- Non-responders are more likely to be:
  - hydropic at commencement of treatment (approximately 60% eventually achieve sinus rhythm)
  - long VA rhythms.
- Hydrops is the main risk factor for death and, in spite of treatment, mortality is:
  - 50% if remains in SVT
  - 10% if SR restored.
- Sudden fetal death can occur while on and even when responding to treatment.
- Survivors who were hydropic have an increased risk of neurodevelopmental problems. Several factors may be contributory:
  - Low cardiac output *in utero*.
  - Prematurity.
  - Coexistent cerebral malformations.
  - Associated syndromes.

Postnatal management

This will be influenced by a number of factors but drug treatment does not need to be continued postnatally if:

- only on 1 drug and
- SR established at least 4 weeks before delivery
- rhythm was AVRT or atrial flutter
- heart is structurally and functionally normal
- all traces of hydrops resolved.

Follow-up may only need to be for 6 months but will be influenced by:

- any symptomatic recurrences in early infancy
- presence of pre-excited ECG (risk of arrhythmias persists).
- need for neurodevelopmental surveillance if hydropic *in utero*
- existence of structural/functional cardiac abnormalities
- coexisting non-cardiac conditions.

There is a small chance of SVT recurrence in later childhood but unless ECG is pre-excited there is no need to follow up because of this. Families should be told to seek medical advice if possible symptoms of SVT occur.

Ventricular tachycardia (VT)

This is much rarer than SVT; some large series of fetal tachycardia have no identified cases.

Diagnosis by echocardiography

- Usually loss of AV synchrony (retrograde VA conduction uncommon).
- Ventricular rate usually faster than atrial.
- Ventricular rate can be <200/min.

Associations

- As for SVT except pre-excitation on postnatal ECG not a feature unless patient has cardiac tumour.
- Congenital long QT syndromes (LQTS) which may show:
    - definite or suggestive family history (most cases are autosomal dominant but recessive inheritance and sporadic cases occur)
    - bradycardia when in SR
    - 2nd- or 3rd-degree heart block *in utero*.

Management

- If congenital LQTS is suspected, discuss with family:
    - ECG on 1st-degree relatives irrespective of symptoms (penetrance varies)
    - Gene testing any relative with abnormal ECG
- Treatment of VT not always needed but probably indicated if:
    - sustained episodes
    - rate >180/min (idioventricular rhythm with rates below this well tolerated in fetus and newborn and often resolve spontaneously)
    - myocardial function depressed
    - ascending aortic Doppler velocity is markedly reduced in VT
    - LQTS strongly suspected
    - intracardiac tumour
    - haemodynamically important structural heart disease.

- Treatment:
  - Check maternal electrolytes including calcium and magnesium.
  - Use maternal replacement therapy if necessary, especially if LQTS suspected.
  - Drugs, see below.
  - Delivery by caesarean section in fetus mature enough in view of potential problems with drug therapy.
- Transplacental drug regimens:
  - Observe the standard precautions as for SVT.
  - Use standard maternal oral doses and monitoring.
  - Beta blockers are postnatal treatment of choice for LQTS. Potential risk is further slowing of sinus rate which may facilitate onset of VT. Extent to which propranolol crosses the placenta is unclear.
  - Amiodarone and flecainide contraindicated in LQTS but may be used for fetal VT from other causes.

Prognosis

- Related to the cause and associations.
- If an underlying cause or association is not found, it may have a self-limiting course.
- If drug treatment given, this may not need to be continued after the newborn period depending on the cause.
- Data from large numbers of cases not available.

Slow abnormal rhythms

Rhythm definition and AV timing are determined by methods already described.

Sinus bradycardia

- Rate <110/min.
- Fetal distress must be excluded.
- If transient can be normal requiring no action (➲ p. 186).
- Shows normal 1:1 AV synchrony.
- Rate varies.
- May be a sign of LQTS:
  - Take detailed family history.
  - Consider parental ECGs.
- Abnormality of cardiac structure or function uncommon but must be ruled out.
- Consider maternal hypothyroidism or drug ingestion.
- Warrants close follow-up for:
  - monitoring fetal well-being
  - other features of LQTS such as AV block or VT
  - postnatal ECG.

Atrioventricular block

AV block is also termed heart block. It is categorized by the ECG relationship between P waves and QRS complexes:

First-degree heart block

- The PR interval is longer than normal. This causes a prolonged AV time on fetal echo, however assessed. Note:
  - To identify this requires considerable skill.
  - It is unknown whether this can be a normal variant, as it can postnatally.
  - It can be transient in maternal collagen vascular diseases.
  - It may herald progression to higher degrees of block.

Second-degree heart block

- Has a number of patterns in all of which atrial signals are not always followed by ventricular ones (Fig. 17.8):
  - It is not clear if this can be normal in the fetus (one form of 2nd-degree block is normal in sleeping children—the Wenckebach phenomenon).
  - Is associated with LQTS.
  - Has a weak association with structural heart lesions.
  - May progress to complete AV block.
  - Is reported reversible by treatment in some circumstances (➲ p. 202).
  - Must be distinguished from blocked atrial ectopics.

Third-degree (complete) heart block (CHB)

- Shows no relationship between the timing of atrial and ventricular activity (Fig. 17.9).

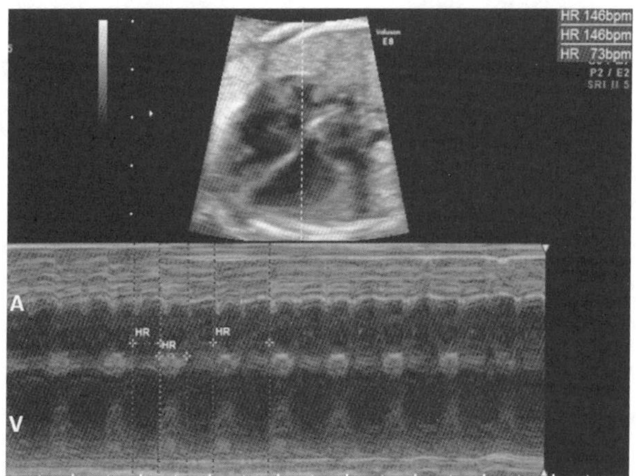

Fig. 17.8 M-mode of 2:1 2nd-degree heart block showing regular atrial contractions (A) with every other one being conducted to ventricles (V) giving a rate of 73/min.

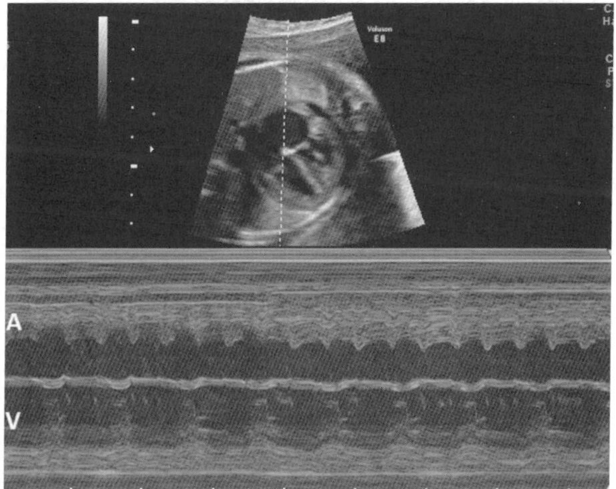

Fig. 17.9 M-mode of complete heart block, there is no consistent relationship between the regular atrial (A) contractions and the ventricular (V) ones which have a rate of 56/min.

Causes and associations of CHB

- Structurally abnormal heart:
  - Often complex (especially congenitally corrected TGA).
  - When found in left atrial isomerism (➔ p. 158), there are usually structural heart disease and non-compacted left ventricular cardiomyopathy in addition.
- Structurally normal heart:
  - There is a strong (>80%) association with maternal anti-SSA/Ro and anti-SSB/La antibodies whether or not the mother has clinical manifestations of Sjögren syndrome, systemic lupus erythematosus, or rheumatoid arthritis. See Box 17.4.
  - If clinically well, an antibody-positive woman may subsequently develop one of these diseases.
  - If a woman has one of these antibodies there is a 2–5% risk of fetal CHB.
  - If a previous pregnancy was affected by antibody-induced CHB, the risk is up to 25% in subsequent pregnancies.
  - Lesser degrees of heart block may be detected in such pregnancies which then progress to CHB (although 1st-degree heart block may resolve).
  - As well as heart block, maternal antibodies may produce cardiomyopathy in the fetus (➔ Chapter 24) and in childhood.
  - The fetal cardiomyopathy can be generalized or focal.
  - Of those without maternal collagen vascular disease or anti-SSA or anti-SSB antibodies, many will have no cause identified but some will turn out to have a LQTS or a cardiomyopathy.

Treatment of CHB without structural heart disease

- Survival after fetal cardiac pacing has yet to be achieved.
- There are reports that maternal steroid therapy can cause improvement in the degree of AV block, although this is not reported in all series.
- There is also evidence that treatment of CHB with steroids improves outcome even if the fetus remains in CHB, presumably as myocarditis independent of rhythm may be of functional significance.
- Thus the use of steroids when there is 2nd- or 3rd-degree heart block in the setting of maternal antibodies is the practice in some centres.
- This approach is not universal as results vary, equivalent outcomes are described with other regimens and steroids have risks for fetus and mother.
- Fetal heart rate can be increased by maternal administration of sympathomimetics (commonly terbutaline) and some groups use this approach if fetal heart rate is <55/min although clear evidence of improved outcome is again debated.
- Some groups reserve steroids and sympathomimetics for fetuses that show evidence of hydrops or severe AV valve regurgitation.
- A management algorithm is given in Box 17.4.

Box 17.4 Fetal heart block associated with maternal antibody

Confirm normal heart structure

Normal fetal health and cardiac function
- 1st-degree AV block—monitor every 7 days, weeks 18 to 28.
- 2nd degree AV block—consider maternal dexamethasone 4 mg daily. Continue if block regresses or does not progress, stop if 3rd-degree AV block develops.
- 3rd degree AV block—monitor every 1 to 2 weeks.

3rd-degree AV block with impaired systolic function/hydrops
- Consider maternal sympathomimetic if rate <55/min.
- Consider maternal dexamethasone.
- Consider delivery for pacing if rate <55/min and if fetal maturity adequate (? >34 weeks).

Prognosis for CHB
- With structural CHD, fetal death occurs in >50% of cases and neonatal/infant outlook is poor.
- Without structural CHD:
  - Hydrops carries a high mortality.
  - Heart rate has not consistently aided prediction of outcome.
  - Falling heart rate is similarly hard to interpret.
- Neonatal pacemaker insertion is likely if:
  - fetal heart rate <50/min
  - hydrops is present
  - fetus has LQTS.

Irregular rhythms

These can be fast, slow, or normal rate. The following need to be considered when an irregular fetal heart rhythm is detected. Fuller details of these conditions are discussed in other topics in this chapter.

- Atrial ectopics (Fig. 17.4):
  - The rate will be slower the higher the number of blocked ectopics.
- Ventricular ectopics (Fig. 17.10):
  - Much rarer than atrial.
- Brief physiological sinus bradycardia:
  - Rate change is often abrupt over less than 5 cardiac cycles.
- Atrial flutter:
  - More commonly is regular but AV conduction ratio may change.
- Chaotic atrial rhythm (multifocal atrial tachycardia) and junctional ectopic tachycardia:
  - Are rare forms of SVT.
  - The most noticeable feature is tachycardia.
  - Rhythm is also irregular although this may not be recognized without detailed analysis.
- Ventricular tachycardia:
  - Rare in the fetus.
  - Usually slightly irregular although this may not be recognized without detailed analysis.

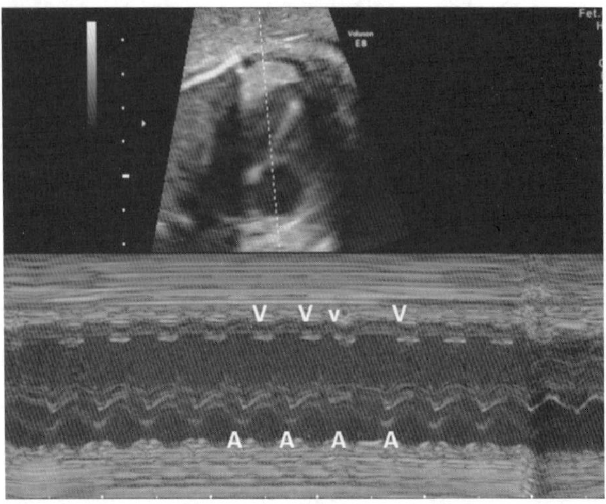

Fig. 17.10 M-mode of SR with atrial contractions (A) preceding ventricular ones (V) then a ventricular ectopic (v) coming prematurely and not preceded by A. There is a compensatory pause before normal AV synchrony is restored.

Chapter 18

Cardiac function

Assessment of cardiac function

Introduction

Fetal echocardiography is used increasingly in the assessment of cardiovascular well-being. Objective assessment of cardiac function can be difficult and subjective observation is often helpful, even if unquantified.

- This chapter will cover simple, reproducible methods to quantify function suitable for use in busy clinical practices.
- Sophisticated and advanced techniques, including the use of speckle tracking, tissue Doppler imaging, 4D, and STIC are beyond the scope of this chapter.
- The purpose of the assessments discussed here is to identify the stressed or failing fetal heart at an early stage and allow monitoring of serial changes
- Cardiac function, if severely compromised, will be associated with general markers of ill health including:
    - pericardial effusion larger than physiological (➔ Chapter 6)
    - hydrops
    - reduced movement.
- Monitoring of heart function is helpful in the management of pregnancies with:
    - fetal hydrops, for whatever cause (➔ Chapter 22)
    - twin–twin transfusion syndrome (➔ Chapter 23)
    - fetal anaemia (➔ Chapter 24)
    - evolving cardiomyopathies (➔ Chapter 19)
    - fetal arrhythmias (➔ Chapter 17)
    - severe intrauterine growth restriction
    - maternal diabetes, especially when control is suboptimal.

The ductus venosus

- The ductus venosus (venous duct) is particularly accessible for interrogation and useful in the assessment of heart function.
- It connects the umbilical vein to the IVC:
    - The DV is a narrow funnel-shaped vessel.
    - Thus blood velocity increases through the vessel.
    - It carries more highly oxygenated blood which does not then pass through the liver.
    - DV blood is preferentially directed by the Eustachian valve in the RA across the foramen ovale to the left atrium.
    - Then to the LV to supply oxygen rich blood to the coronary circulation and brain.
- The DV can be visualized on 2D imaging and is then confirmed with colour Doppler as flow is accelerating through the vessel.
- PW Doppler can then be used to analyse the wave form.
- Flow should always be anterograde towards the heart, even in atrial systole (Fig. 18.1).
- A waves, occurring with RA contraction, will be identifiable as a trough but this should not reach the baseline or be reversed.
- An abnormal wave form in the DV is similar to the normal wave form in the hepatic vessels emphasizing the importance of defining the anatomy with a good 2D image before using colour or PW Doppler.
- The wave form cannot be interpreted if the fetus is breathing or rhythm is not SR.

- Retrograde flow in atrial systole is never normal and may be due to abnormalities of:
  - cardiac anatomy
  - cardiac function
  - venous anatomy
  - placental resistance.

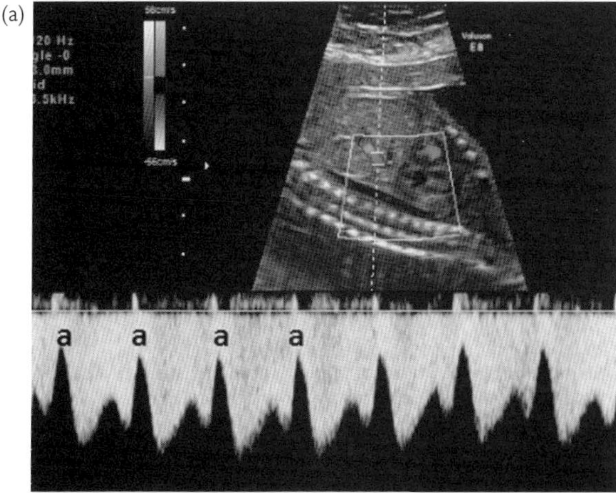

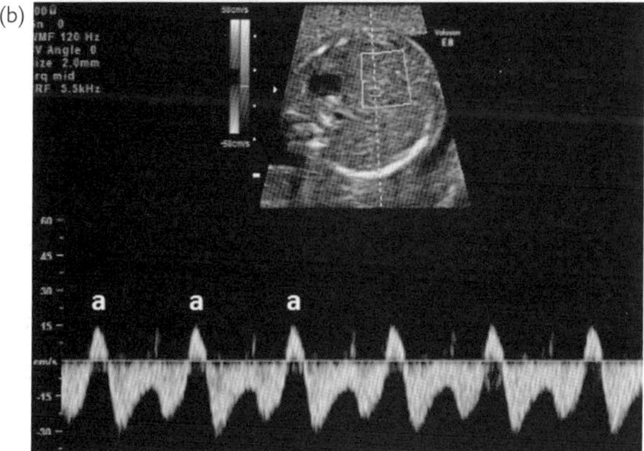

Fig. 18.1 Ductus venosus PW Doppler signal with flow towards heart being away from transducer. (a) Normal showing effect of atrial contraction on reduction of velocity. (b) Abnormal with reversal of a wave (in this case due to severe cardiomyopathy).

General methods

Heart size

- The fetal heart should occupy ⅓ of the chest.
- Measuring the circumference of the heart on a cross-sectional image of the fetal chest and comparing it to the chest circumference gives a cardiothoracic ratio (C:T ratio):
  - Normal value is <0.5.
- These measurements can be used to calculate a heart:chest area ratio:
  - Normal value is 0.2–0.35 (Fig. 18.2).
- The following points are relevant:
  - A symmetrical section of the chest must be obtained.
  - Changes over time are more important than a single measurement.
- If only one heart chamber is enlarged, interpretation of changes in size depends on the aetiology and may not necessarily reflect global cardiac function or status.
- Pericardial fluid can be included as long as this is clearly specified, and depth of fluid documented.
- A small heart is also associated with a guarded prognosis.

Contractility

- Often a subjective impression will suffice but accurate measurements can be obtained using 4-chamber, long- or short-axis views in 2D or M-mode (Fig. 6.4).
- Ejection fraction or fractional shortening can then be calculated and repeated serial measurements used to monitor changes.

Atrioventricular valve regurgitation

- Physiological tricuspid valve regurgitation is common, especially with optimum scanning conditions and is a normal variant.
- Mitral regurgitation is not considered a normal finding.
- Quantifying TR may be difficult but incudes:
  - duration of TR jet within the cardiac cycle
  - size of jet, length (should not extend more than ⅓ into RA), and breadth
  - may be described as trivial/ physiological, mild, moderate, or severe.
- Sequential reduction in the velocity of AV valve regurgitation suggests worsening ventricular function.

Atrioventricular valve inflow patterns

- Disturbance to diastolic function will be reflected by changes to inflow patterns, E:A wave morphology.
- In early gestation, the E (passive) wave is smaller than the A (atrial contraction) wave as fetal myocardium is less compliant than postnatally (Fig. 6.4).
- As gestation advances, compliance increases and the size of the E wave increases to be equal to the size A wave by term.
- Monophasic inflow (fusion of E and a waves) suggests significant diastolic dysfunction.
- Diastolic dysfunction, as seen in twin–twin transfusion syndrome, may be an early warning sign.

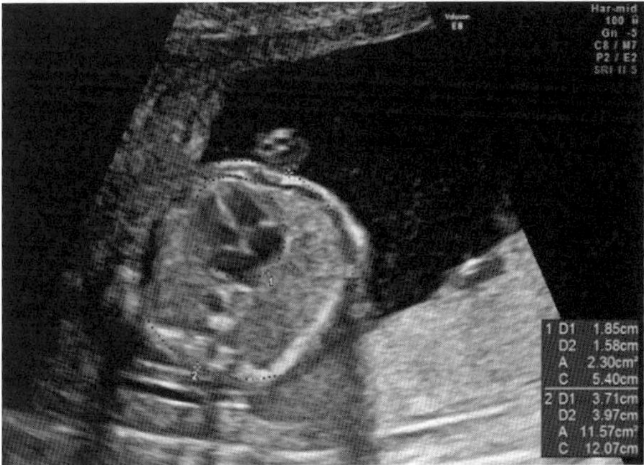

Fig. 18.2 4-chamber view with measurement of heart (1) and chest (2) ellipse diameters (D1, D2) and circumference (C) with calculation of area (A) of each allowing ratios for both to be determined.

Myocardial performance score (Tei Index)

- This is a Doppler-derived score which is obtained using PW Doppler assessment of inflow and outflow blood velocity signals from both the LV and (slightly harder technically) the RV.
- This score reflects global myocardial performance by assessing duration of flow through the AV valves and outflow tracts:
  - Is not altered by heart rate.
  - Remains constant throughout gestation.
  - Reflects both systolic and diastolic function.
  - Normal value should be around 0.36 (0.28–0.44).
  - An increased score suggests a reduction in function.
- It requires plenty of practice to obtain consistent and reliable results.
- It can be time-consuming.
- For detailed information search literature.

Cardiovascular profile score

- The cardiovascular profile score can be used for serial assessment and to help with prediction of outcome.
  - Changes in the cardiovascular profile score may occur before the onset of terminal decompensation.
- Details of the score are given in Table 18.1:
  - Lower scores are associated with worse outcomes.
  - Falling scores are particularly worrying.

Table 18.1 Heart failure score—cardiovascular profile score*

	2 points	1 point	0 points
Hydrops	None	Ascites or pleural or pericardial effusion	Skin oedema
Doppler			
• umbilical vein	Normal	Normal	Pulsatile
• ductus venosus	Normal	Any retrograde signal in atrial systole	–
CTR (heart/ chest area)	0.2–0.35	0.35–0.50	>0.5 or <0.2
Function	No AV regurgitation	Pansystolic TR	Pansystolic MR
	RV and LV FS >0.28	RV or LV FS <0.28	Monophasic AV valve Doppler
	Biphasic AV valve Doppler	–	–
Umbilical artery Doppler	Normal	Absent end-diastolic flow	Reversed end diastolic flow

CTR, cardiothoracic ratio; FC, fractional shortening.

*Adapted from Huhta JC (2005) Fetal congestive heart failure, *Seminars in Fetal & Neonatal Medicine* 10;542–52 with permission from Elsevier.

Chapter 19

Heart muscle disease

Introduction

- Heart muscle disease presenting in the fetus is rare.
- The distinction between myocarditis and non-inflammatory cardiomyopathy is not clear cut and the term cardiomyopathy tends to be used for both categories.
- Primary cardiomyopathy:
  - is often genetically determined although the gene is not always identified
  - may be associated with structural CHD insufficiently severe to impair heart function.
- Secondary heart muscle disease:
  - can be the consequence of fetal illness (e.g. twin–twin transfusion syndrome)
  - can be the result of maternal disease (e.g. maternal infection or antibodies)
  - is seen in severe structural lesions (e.g. PA, IVS, severe AS) and is not discussed further here.
- In the following discussion, it is assumed that cardiac anatomy is normal.
- Fetal cardiomyopathy:
  - Can affect either or both ventricles.
  - Tends to progress during pregnancy.
  - May prevent the fetus from reaching a viable gestation.
- In the following descriptions, it is assumed that cardiac anatomy is normal.
- The commonest cause of fetal cardiomyopathy is idiopathic.
- Prognosis depends on aetiology but is commonly poor.

Types of cardiomyopathy

Cardiomyopathies can be classified in as follows
- Hypertrophic
- Dilated
- Restrictive
- Miscellaneous.

Hypertrophic cardiomyopathy (HCM)

- Recognized by the presence of abnormal hypertrophy of either/both ventricles and/or ventricular septum usually resulting in cardiomegaly (Fig. 19.1).
- Tends to progress during the pregnancy such that function may be impaired and hydrops may develop.

Causes include:
- Autosomal dominant conditions.
- A small proportion of new mutations.
- In about 50% of familial cases a gene may be identifiable.
- If a parent has classic familial autosomal dominant HCM, fetal scanning is not recommended
  - The phenotype very rarely expresses itself prenatally or in the first few post-natal years
  - thus cannot be excluded in the fetus

Other causes include:
- Maternal diabetes:
  - Reflects fetal hyperinsulinism in 3rd trimester.
  - May affect ventricular septum and RV more than LV (Fig. 24.3).
  - Not considered as an indication to rescan in later pregnancy.
  - Rarely clinically important (➲ Chapter 24).
  - More likely if control is suboptimal.
  - Resolves during the first year of postnatal life.
- Recipient twin in twin–twin transfusion syndrome (➲ Chapter 23).
- Noonan's syndrome:
  - In approximately 20%.
  - Most commonly affects the ventricular septum.
  - Pulmonary valve abnormalities may develop in the 3rd trimester.
  - May become haemodynamically significant but rarely in the fetus.
- Some metabolic and storage disorders:
  - Specialist knowledge of diagnostic tests and their application in pregnancy should be sought.

Dilated cardiomyopathy (DCM)

- Dilatation of one or both ventricles, often with thin heart muscle, usually with cardiomegaly (Fig. 19.2):
  - Usually with severe AV valve regurgitation.
  - Usually with poor systolic function with the risk for hydrops.

(a)
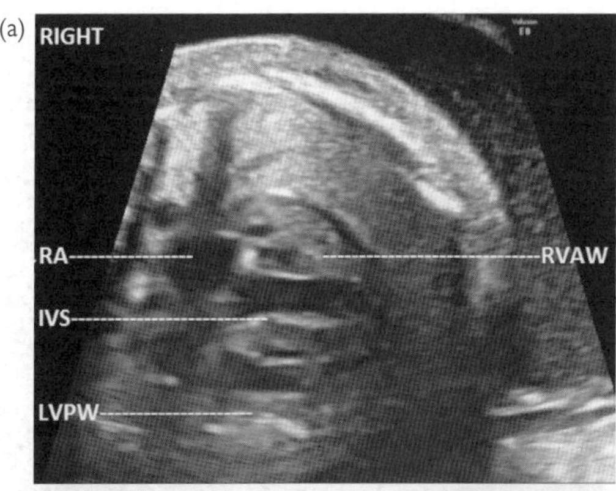

(b)
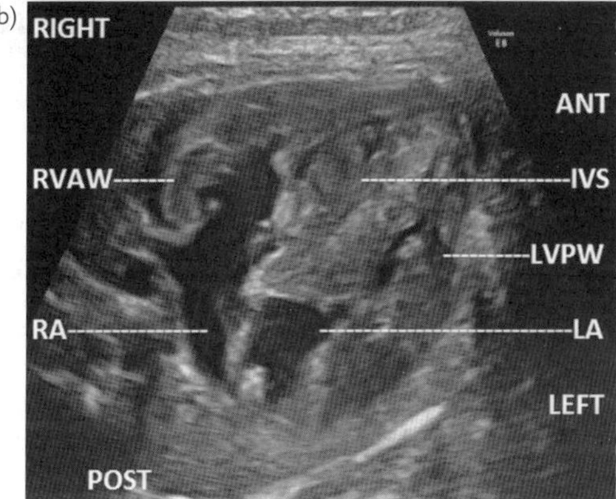

Fig. 19.1 (a) 4-chamber view showing generalized hypertrophy. Recipient in twin–twin transfusion syndrome. (b) 4-chamber view in ventricular diastole showing gross generalized hypertrophy. No cause identified.

Causes include:

- Familial (DCM) which may be autosomal dominant.
- Some metabolic disorders.
- Sustained fetal arrhythmias, especially tachycardias.
- Fetal anaemia after initial hyperdynamic phase.
- Fetal AV malformation after initial hyperdynamic phase.
- Fetal infection in particular parvovirus which can cause:
    - anaemia
    - myocarditis.

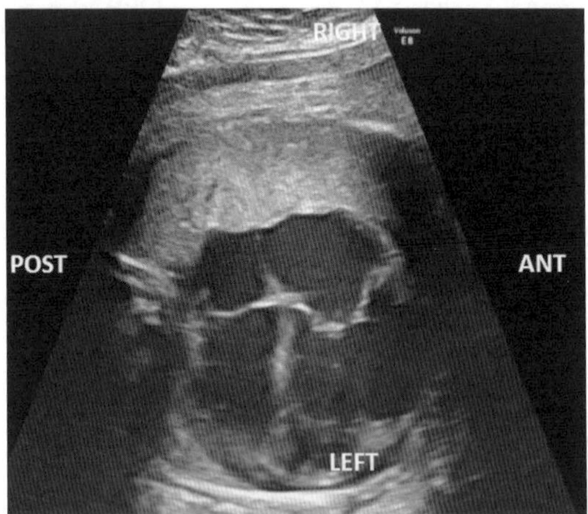

Fig. 19.2 4-chamber view showing grossly enlarged heart in ventricular systole. DCM cause unidentified.

Restrictive cardiomyopathy

- Very rare in the fetus, usually with a genetic cause so that the recurrence risk may be high.
- Recognized on imaging by enlargement of the atria with preserved ventricular systolic function (Fig. 19.3).
- Usually poorly tolerated with onset of hydrops in the 2nd trimester.

Miscellaneous

Some hearts fit into more than one of the above-mentioned categories anatomically and haemodynamically and may evolve from one to another over time. Diseases to consider with unusual cardiomyopathies include:

- maternal anti-Ro antibodies:
  - myocardium may be echogenic with areas resembling endocardial fibroelastosis (Fig. 19.4).
- viral causes which may be transient
- aneuploidies or abnormal microarray results
- left atrial isomerism (➔ Chapter 14) is associated with non-compaction which is otherwise rare in the fetus.

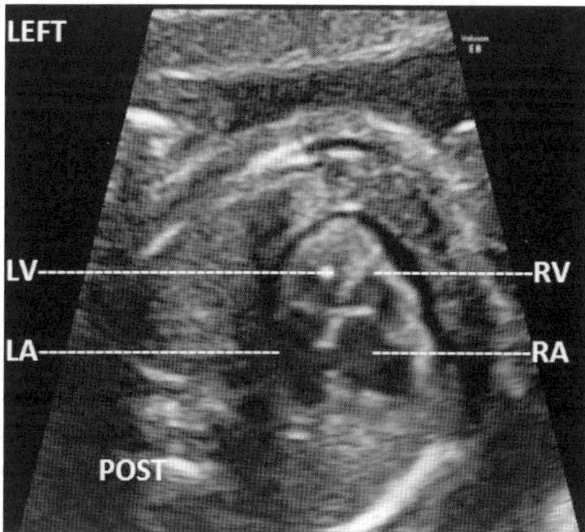

Fig. 19.3 4-chamber view in ventricular systole in RCM showing atria larger than ventricles ('ice cream cone').

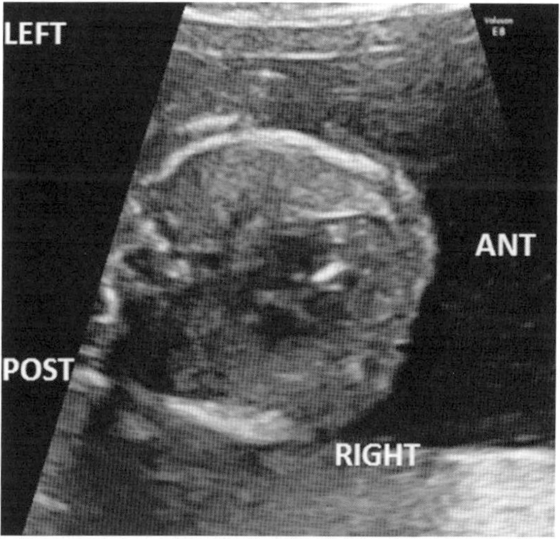

Fig. 19.4 4-chamber view showing echobright areas in IVS and possibly LV posterior wall. Presumed maternal systemic lupus erythematosus.

Assessment

Assessment of heart function is discussed in ➲ Chapter 18. Heart muscle thickness can be measured using:

- 2D imaging
- M-mode
- short-axis, long-axis, or 4-chamber views

Normal ventricular and septal myocardial thickness should not exceed 5mm in the last trimester.

Treatment

- Treatment involves correcting the underlying cause if identified and if possible.
- Drug treatment is unproven except in the cases of fetal tachycardias although there is some evidence that digoxin may be of value even in sinus rhythm.
- Steroid medication is used by some in maternal antibody-related heart muscle disease if systolic function is poor or AV valve regurgitation is severe as well as for heart block (➲ Chapter 24).

Chapter 20

Cardiac tumours

Introduction

- Cardiac tumours are rare.
- Single or multiple tumours can exist and detailed assessment of number, size, and site is essential as a reference point for subsequent evaluation.
- An assessment of the echogenicity is appropriate (homogeneous/heterogeneous/cystic).
- Identification requires subsequent monitoring for:
  - fetal well-being
  - growth of the tumour (s)
  - planning management of delivery and neonatal period.
- It is important to consider non-cardiac associations.
- Most tumours increase in size during pregnancy and are rarely identified before 20 weeks' gestation.
- Some present as an incidental finding at a growth scan; others are discovered during a more detailed assessment of:
  - cardiac arrhythmia
  - pericardial effusion
  - hydrops.
- Tumours can originate from any part of the heart including:
  - myocardium
  - pericardium
  - endocardium.
- Most are histologically benign and prognosis is dependent on the haemodynamic impact of the tumour and on any associated non-cardiac problems.
- Echocardiography can define most of the useful information although in some the differential diagnosis is difficult and further investigation by MRI (cardiac or cranial) may be used if doubt exists.
- Haemodynamic effects depend on the position, number, and size of tumours and include:
  - interference with myocardial function
  - obstruction to forward flow through a valve causing hypoplasia of affected chambers or vessels
  - valvar regurgitation
  - arrhythmias including benign atrial ectopic beats, SVT, and ventricular arrhythmias causing sudden intrauterine death.
- Serial assessment of cardiac function and rhythm is appropriate once viability is reached.
- For a very few cases, early delivery and possible neonatal surgery may be required.
- Sometimes cardiac tumours are the initial manifestation of a genetic syndrome with significant implications for wider issues and the value of parental/sibling assessment and of genetic testing needs to be considered.
- Echogenic foci ('golf balls') are recognized normal variants but occasionally cannot be differentiated from pathological tumours (➔ p. 222).

- Although all tumours are rare, the following are recognized *in utero* in order of decreasing frequency:
  - rhabdomyoma
  - teratoma
  - fibroma
  - haemangioma (exceedingly rare)
  - myxoma (exceedingly rare).

Echogenic foci

- Often termed 'golf balls' (Fig. 20.1).
- Are a normal variant.
- Have no haemodynamic significance.
- Echodense homogeneous circular regions most often in the papillary muscles of the left ventricle.
- Can be seen in right ventricle.
- Unlike pathological tumours they are rare in the atria.
- Up to 5 mm in diameter.
- Pathology poorly described because of natural history, are thought to contain calcium.
- May be single, less commonly multiple.
- Most commonly detected at anomaly scan.
- Usually gone or much smaller by term in contrast to pathological tumours.
- If confidently diagnosed do not need further investigation or follow-up in pregnancy or afterwards.
- If doubt exists about their nature, they should be monitored until innocence is assured or a tumour of a pathological nature is apparent.
- Association with chromosomal abnormality is unclear but when first detected a careful search for other 'soft markers' is advised although formal screening test results are more important.

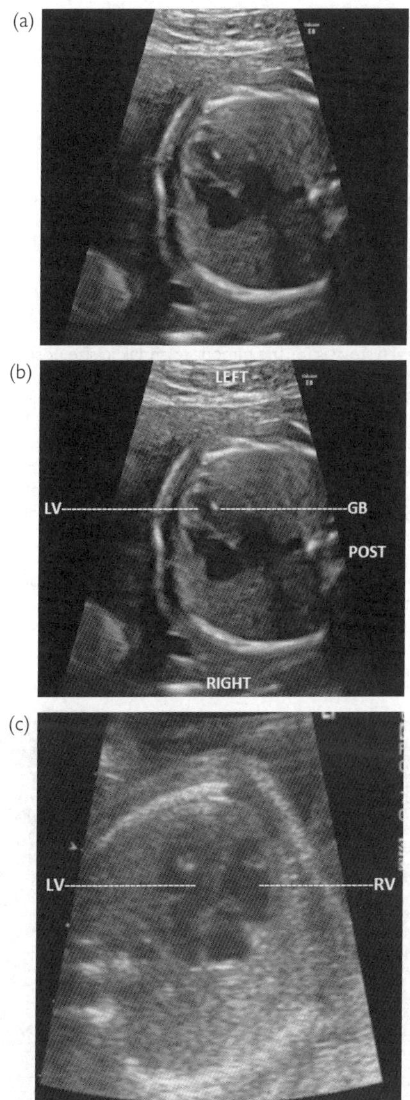

Fig. 20.1 4-chamber view showing single echodense region in LV cavity—a 'golf ball', (a) plain, (b) annotated. (c) 4-chamber view showing echodense lesions in both LV and RV, multiple 'golf balls'.

Rhabdomyoma

- The commonest fetal cardiac tumour, representing around 80% of tumours seen prenatally.
- Histologically they are a form of hamartoma—an overgrowth of tissue normally present at the site of origin.
- On ultrasound they are well-defined, homogeneous echogenic masses in the atrial or ventricular wall or in the ventricular septum.
- Usually become apparent between 20 and 30 weeks' gestation, occasionally earlier.
- May initially appear as a single tumour but in most cases, multiple tumours become identifiable in time (Fig. 20.2).
- Although benign they grow during pregnancy, probably under the influence of maternal hormones and, depending on their position in the heart, can have significant haemodynamic effects.
- The natural history is for the tumour to shrink in size postnatally and thus surgical intervention is rarely indicated.
- Around 80% of fetuses with multiple rhabdomyomata will have tuberose sclerosis, a syndrome which:
    - is a dominantly inherited disorder but usually appears as a new mutation
    - *TSC1* (25%) or *TSC2* (65%) gene mutations are detected in 90% of postnatal cases of TS with 10% having no known mutation
    - genotype–phenotype correlations are not yet well enough delineated to predict prognosis for use in prenatal counselling
    - is variable in terms of its impact on quality of life
    - may be associated with intracerebral tumours, some of which may be detectable prenatally with MRI
    - is not excluded by the absence of cerebral tumours as these may not develop until later in life
    - renal tumours are unlikely to be detected in the fetus

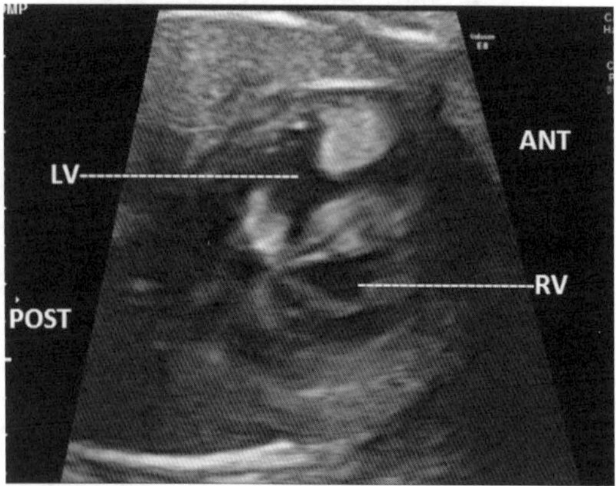

Fig. 20.2 4-chamber view showing multiple intracardiac tumours (IVS, LV, AV valve). Rhabdomyomata.

Teratoma

- Teratomas are usually single, arise from the pericardium, and are often associated with a pericardial effusion (Fig. 20.3).
- Very rarely they are intracardiac.
- In contrast to rhabdomyomas, teratomas are of mixed echogenicity with cystic areas as well as areas of calcification.
- Usually identified at around 20 weeks' gestation and grow through pregnancy.
- By compromising systemic venous return to the heart and blood flow through the heart, teratomas are more likely to cause significant haemodynamic disturbance and may result in chamber hypoplasia.
- Drainage of a large pericardial effusion may be indicated if tamponade is likely and to prevent progression of hydrops.
- Recurrence of effusion is common and resection of tumour has been attempted *in utero*.
- Postnatal surgery is usually successful depending on gestation, cardiac growth, and well-being at delivery.

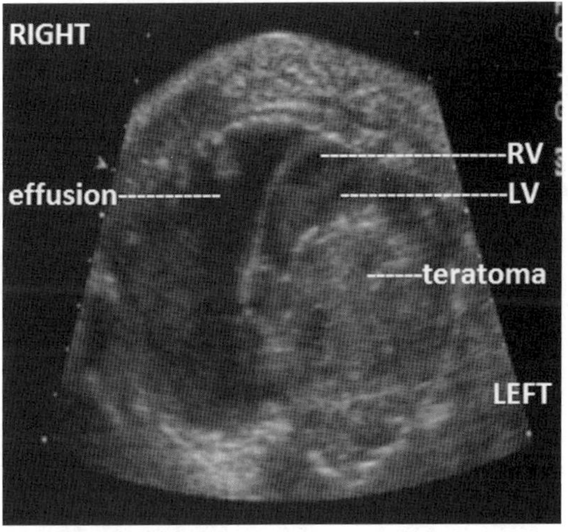

Fig. 20.3 4-chamber view showing very large teratoma posterior to LA resulting in a massive pericardial effusion and diminutive left heart.

Fibroma

- Benign and usually solitary.
- Develop in the ventricular wall myocardium or septum.
- May be of uniform echogenicity and thus hard to distinguish from rhabdomyoma.
- Some degenerate and thus appear partly cystic and with areas of calcification.
- Postnatally they tend to continue to grow and require surgical resection, especially if symptomatic or associated with arrhythmias.

Haemangioma

- Extremely rare in the fetus.
- Usually of mixed echogenicity and although vascular, the vessels are too small to define with colour Doppler.
- Tend to arise from the base of the heart adjacent to the right atrium and may extend into the right atrium.
- May be associated with a pericardial effusion and hydrops.
- Usually successfully surgically removed postnatally.

Myxoma

- A benign tumour which is extremely rare in the fetus.
- There can be a family history of cardiac myxoma (including an association with Carney syndrome).
- Usually echogenic and pedunculated and thus mobile and may move across valves.

Chapter 21

Nuchal translucency and the heart

Introduction

- Nuchal screening is performed between 11+0 and 13+6 weeks and offered routinely to all pregnant women.
- The primary objective is to identify fetuses at increased risk for a chromosomal anomaly:
  - Used in combination with maternal serum biochemical markers.
- Increased measurements are associated with increased risk of chromosomal abnormality and of major structural anomalies.
- Fetuses with increased nuchal translucency (NT) have an increased risk for CHD:
  - Even if the karyotype or non-invasive prenatal testing result (➔ Chapter 8) are normal.
- This risk increases with increasing NT measurements for all types of CHD.
- Evidence of cardiac dysfunction might alert to the presence of a structural anomaly:
  - TR
  - Abnormal waveform in the ductus venosus (➔ Chapter 18).

The nuchal scan

- The nuchal area is measured to the nearest 1/10th mm using standardized methods:
  - Readily achievable by experienced operators with a high degree of reproducibility.
- Some major structural fetal anomalies, including cardiac anomalies, may also be identified during this scan

The nuchal scan and the heart

- The mechanism of increased NT with cardiac anomalies is unclear.
- Risk of CHD and NT centiles are listed in Table 21.1.
- Risk of CHD with NT measurements are listed in Table 21.2.
- Not all fetuses with CHD have increased nuchal measurements.
- Most fetuses with increased NT and a normal karyotype have normal hearts.
- Up to 50% of fetuses with major structural CHD have increased NT.
- The value of NT measurement in screening for CHD is unproven.

Table 21.1 NT centile and approximate risk of CHD with normal karyotype

Nuchal centile	Risk of CHD (%)
Median–95th	<1
95th–99th	1.8
>99th	3.5–12.6

Table 21.2 NT measurement and approximate risk of CHD with normal karyotype

Nuchal measurement (mm)	Risk of CHD (%)
3.5–4.4	3.5
4.5–5.4	6.4
5.5+	12.7

Management

- An increased NT of >3.5mm is an indication for detailed echocardiography; we recommend:
  - an early assessment at 14–16 weeks
  - repeated at 20–22 weeks even if earlier scan normal.
- Fetuses with increased NT, normal karyotype, normal anomaly, and cardiac scans usually have a good outcome.

Chapter 22

Hydrops and the heart

Introduction

Hydrops fetalis refers to the pathological condition where fluid collects in 2 or more body cavities; it represents excessive accumulation of interstitial fluid, initially in the serous spaces (pericardial, pleural, and peritoneal cavities, see Figs 22.1, 22.2, and 22.3) but in time may progress to generalized skin oedema (Fig. 22.4). It is the common pathway for many different disease processes.

Hydrops is the consequence of fetal cardiovascular decompensation; the cause may be cardiac or non-cardiac in origin. Its onset represents cardiac failure for whatever reason and it is associated with inadequate tissue perfusion. Fetal hydrops is associated with a high morbidity and mortality pre- and postnatally.

- Predicting survival remains a challenge.
- Antenatal treatment is only possible for a few specific causes.
- Echocardiography has an important role in:
  - identifying a cause
  - quantifying haemodynamic involvement
  - monitoring progression
  - monitoring response to treatment when relevant
- The effect of hydrops on cerebral perfusion remains undefined.

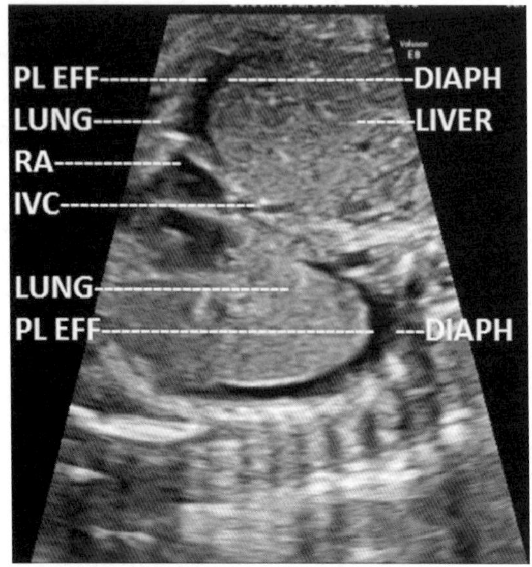

Fig. 22.1 Oblique long-axis view showing bilateral pleural effusions (PL EFF).

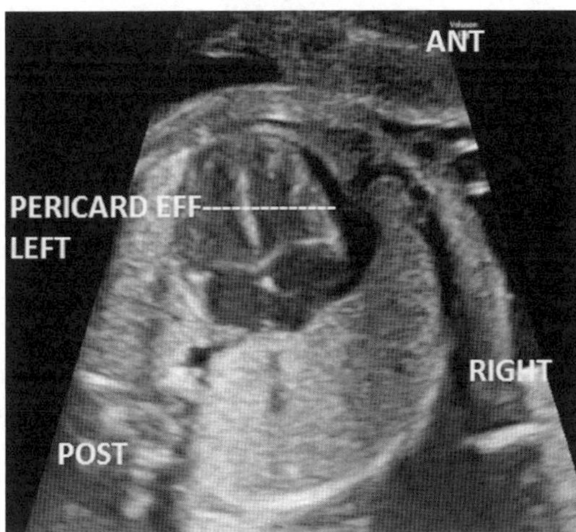

Fig. 22.2 4-chamber view showing anterior pericardial effusion.

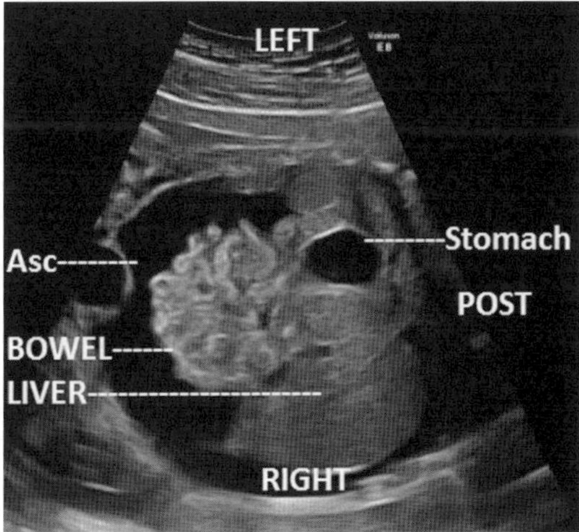

Fig. 22.3 Short-axis view of abdomen showing bowel surrounded by ascitic fluid.

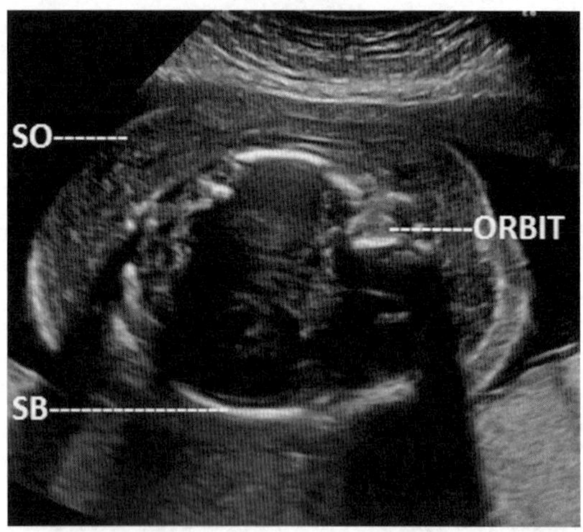

Fig. 22.4 Coronal view of skull showing large amount of oedema (SO) between bone (SB) and skin.

Pathophysiology of hydrops

- The RV handles ⅔ of combined cardiac output in the normal fetus.
- The infrastructure of the RV is such that, in comparison to the LV, it:
    - is more compliant
    - generates less force
    - is less resistant to increases in cardiac load
    - is more susceptible to failure.
- Small increases in systemic venous pressures results in:
    - increased extravascular shift
    - reduction in circulating volume
    - reduced combined cardiac output
    - development of hydrops.
- If progressive this causes:
    - low tissue perfusion
    - progressive acidosis
    - fetal death.
- This series of complex interactions can be triggered by many different pathologies producing the final expression of hydrops.
- Cardiac output is determined by heart rate and stroke volume.
- There is little scope for increased heart rate in the fetus.
- Stroke volume is determined by:
    - preload (ventricular myocardial stretching in diastole)
    - ventricular myocardial performance
    - afterload.

Preload

Influenced by various factors including:

- anaemia
- TTTS
- systemic AV malformations
- pericardial effusion/other intrathoracic space-occupying lesion
- atrial dysfunction—impaired in atrial arrhythmias.

Ventricular myocardial performance

- Dysfunction can be:
    - diastolic—inability to relax normally thus reducing ventricular filling, or
    - systolic—inability to pump normally thus reducing volume ejected.

May be caused by:

- Heart muscle disease:
    - cardiomyopathies
    - myocarditis.
- Some structural cardiac lesions:
    - Ebstein's anomaly
    - aortic stenosis.

Afterload

Determined by systemic vascular resistance which increases in:

- hypertension, as in the recipient twin in TTTS
- placental dysfunction

Aetiology

- In many cases the aetiology of hydrops is never determined.
- Viral infections are a common cause.
- Many different fetal anomalies may be responsible; some of the more common causes are summarized in Table 22.1.

Table 22.1 Causes of fetal hydrops

		Prenatal treatment possible
Structural CHD	Ebstein's anomaly	+/−
	Severe/critical aortic stenosis	+/−
	Complete AVSD	−
	Premature closure of ductus arteriosus	+/−
	Agenesis of the ductus venosus	−
Arrhythmias	Tachycardia (SVT, flutter)	+
	Bradycardia (complete heart block)	+/−
Cardiomyopathies	See ➲ Chapter 19	+/−
Myocarditis	Including with maternal anti-Ro antibodies	+/−
Cardiac tumours	See ➲ Chapter 20	+/−
Chromosomal	Trisomy 21	−
	Turner syndrome	−
	Triploidy	−
	Rare variants	−
Twin pregnancies	Recipient or less often donor in TTTS (➲ Chapter 23)	+
	Pump twin in TRAP sequence (➲ Chapter 23)	+
Syndromes	Noonan syndrome	−
Non-cardiac structural anomalies	Pleural effusions	+/−
	Congenital diaphragmatic hernia	+/−
	Cystadenomatous malformations	+/−
	Teratoma	+/−
	Arteriovenous fistulae	+/−
	Placental chorioangioma	+/−
Fetal anaemia	Any cause	+/−
Infection	Parvovirus (anaemia and myocarditis)	+
	Cytomegalovirus	−
	Adenovirus	−
	Other	−
Maternal causes	Severe anaemia	+
Unidentified	Commonest group	−

Assessment and monitoring

In the presence of hydrops and as part of the search for an underlying cause, detailed examination should include the following:

- General assessment of:
    - fetal and placental anatomy
    - severity of hydrops
    - fetal biophysical profile.
- From the cardiac perspective, the examination should involve assessment of:
    - cardiac anatomy
    - cardiac size (C:T ratio, see Fig. 18.2)
    - function as discussed in ➡ Chapter 18
    - rhythm (➡ Chapter 17).
- Assessment of the cardiovascular profile score (➡ Chapter 18):
    - more useful than measuring fluid volumes
    - predictive value depends on the underlying cause of hydrops.

Management

- Treatment of underlying pathology may be possible, as in:
  - fetal anaemia
  - fetal tachycardia (response to treatment takes longer in the hydropic fetus)
  - TTTS.
- In the majority of cases management involves:
  - serial monitoring
  - use of steroids in anticipation of premature delivery
  - consideration of early delivery if deterioration occurs at a viable gestation.
- Use of specific drugs to try to improve the fetal well-being is subject for debate but includes:
  - digoxin to improve cardiac function even in sinus rhythm
  - sympathomimetic agents to increase heart rate in heart block (➲ Chapter 17)
  - steroids for possible autoimmune myocarditis (➲ Chapters 17 and 24)
- Maternal well-being must be closely monitored as:
  - maternal disease may be the cause of the hydrops
  - women with hydropic fetuses are at risk of severe pre-eclampsia (mirror syndrome).

Chapter 23

Twins and the heart

Introduction

- Twins account for approximately 2% of all pregnancies.
- Two-thirds of these are dizygotic (DZ)—non-identical twins resulting from fertilization of 2 separate oocytes.
- All DZ twins are dichorionic (DC) and diamniotic.
- The remaining third are monozygotic (MZ)—identical twins, the result of division of a single embryonic cell mass after fertilization.
- MZ twins may be DC diamniotic, monochorionic (MC) diamniotic or MC monoamniotic; very rarely they are conjoined.
- Chorionicity depends on timing of division of the embryonic mass (Table 23.1).
- 7–10% of DC twins will be MZ and therefore identical:
  - A fact not always appreciated postnatally.
  - Zygosity can only be defined non-invasively antenatally if the twins are different sexes.
- Chorionicity refers to the type of placentation and determines the risk to the pregnancy:
  - Chorionicity can be defined on ultrasound antenatally (Fig. 23.1).
- DC twins are not at increased risk for functional cardiac anomalies as they have separate placentas.
- The risk for both structural and functional heart disease in MC twins is increased.
- Intertwin transfusion occurs in the majority of MC twins as a result of placental anastomoses:
  - With the potential for uneven volume distribution
  - The basis of TTTS
  - With an important impact on the cardiovascular systems of both twins.

Table 23.1 Timing of division and type of monozygotic twin

Twin type	DC/diamniotic	MC/diamniotic	MC/monoamniotic	Conjoined
Timing of division of embryonic mass post fertilization	<3 days	3–9 days	9–12 days	Incomplete
Proportion of MZ twins	33%	65%	2%	very rare

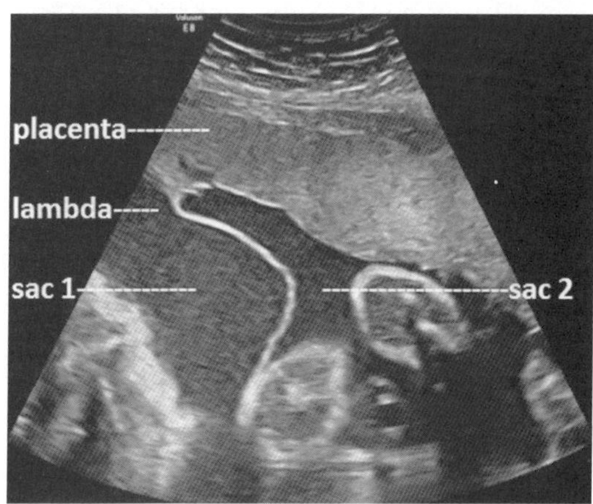

Fig. 23.1 Lambda sign formed by membrane between sacs of DC diamniotic twins meeting the placenta.

Antenatal identification of twin type

- DC twins have:
  - 2 separate placentas
  - 2 layers of chorion and 2 layers of amnion
  - can be diagnosed by defining a lambda sign formed by the thick chorionic membranes (Figs 23.1 and 23.2).
- DC twins are not considered to be at increased risk for cardiac disease although:
  - risk for structural CHD in MZ diamniotic twins is yet to be quantified accurately.
- MC twins can be diamniotic or monoamniotic.
- Monoamniotic DC twins:
  - 1 single placenta in 2 separate sacs
  - 2 separate amnions
  - Thin dividing membrane—T sign (Fig. 23.2).
  - Usually have placental anastomoses and share a circulation.
- Monoamniotic MC twins share a sac such that:
  - there is no dividing membrane
  - umbilical cord entanglement is always present.
- Conjoined twins are extremely rare:
  - Division of the cell mass is incomplete.
  - There is usually cardiac involvement.
- The later the division of the fertilized call mass, the:
  - higher the risk for cardiac anomalies in one or both twins
  - greater the risk for pregnancy complications.

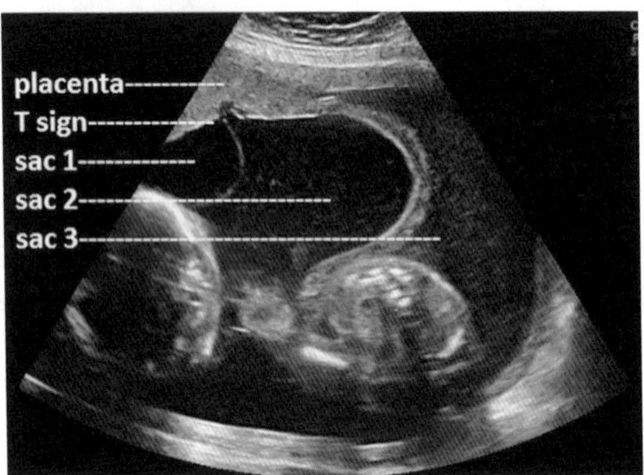

Fig. 23.2 Triplet pregnancy consisting of MC diamniotic twins with thin amniotic membrane separating sacs 1 and 2 and a DC diamniotic fetus (in sac 3) separated by a thick chorionic and amniotic membrane from the MC pair.

Cardiac aspects of monochorionic twins

- MC twins are at an increased risk for cardiac complications.
- This includes structural anomalies:
  - 'Primary'.
  - 'Acquired' as a result of functional complications of TTTS.
- In addition, there are functional anomalies as a consequence of TTTS.

'Primary' structural cardiac lesions

- The risk for at least one of a MC/diamniotic twin pair having structural CHD is between 4% and 11%, even in the absence of TTTS.
- If one MC/diamniotic twin has structural CHD there is an approximate 20% risk that the other will also have CHD.
- If both twins have CHD, the lesions are usually discordant:
  - Even though they are genetically identical.
  - Explained in terms of postzygotic events.
- All forms of CHD are recognized in these fetuses:
  - VSDs are commonest.
- For MA twins the risk is higher:
  - Including for laterality defects which are otherwise uncommon.

'Acquired' cardiac anomalies

- As a consequence of fetal haemodynamics in TTTS.

Twin–twin transfusion syndrome in monochorionic twins

- Intertwin transfusion is virtually always present:
  - As a result of vascular anastomoses in the single placenta.
- TTTS develops in 10–15% of MC/diamniotic twins.
- Cardiovascular abnormalities provide a significant contribution to the high morbidity and mortality in untreated or advanced TTTS.
- There is a well-established method of defining the severity of TTTS according to Quintero staging, see Table 23.2.
- For the majority of MC twins, flow is balanced with even distribution to each twin and thus there:
  - are equal circulating volumes
  - is no disruption to haemodynamics.
- In TTTS, there is unequal volume distribution.
- The recipient twin becomes hypervolaemic and hypertensive, with the potential to cause:
  - cardiac hypertrophy and dilatation
  - AV valve regurgitation
  - diastolic and systolic dysfunction
  - right ventricular outflow tract obstruction
  - hydrops and fetal death.
- The recipient produces natriuretic peptides causing polyuria and thus polyhydramnios.
- The donor twin is hypovolaemic and produces vasoactive agents:
  - increasing vascular resistance in fetus and placenta.
- The donor becomes oliguric with oligohydramnios.

Table 23.2 Quintero staging for twin–twin transfusion syndrome*

Stage I	Donor bladder visible
Stage II	No donor bladder Normal Doppler assessments
Stage III	Abnormal Doppler assessments *For donor:* AEDF/REDF in donor umbilical artery +/− *For recipient:* Abnormal DV flow Pulsatile umbilical vein
Stage IV	Hydrops in 1 twin
Stage V	Death of 1/both twins

AEDF, absent end-diastolic flow; DV, ductus venosus; REDF, reversed end-diastolic flow.

* Adapted with permission from Macmillan Publishers Ltd: *Journal of Perinatology* 19:550–555, Quintero R.A et al Staging of Twin-Twin Transfusion Syndrome, copyright 1999.

- As a result of their shared circulation:
  - each is subjected to the other's circulating vasoactive agents
  - which might further aggravate the situation
  - the well-being of one twin critically depends on that of the other.
- Cardiac manifestations of TTTS are detectable early in the disease process and can be useful in helping:
  - guide management in association with Quintero staging
  - assess response to treatment.
- Treatment of TTTS involves laser coagulation of the anastomoses:
  - effectively creating a DC placenta
  - thus terminating the TTTS process
  - and allowing the cardiac anomalies to regress.
- Acquired structural cardiac anomalies include:
  - right ventricular outflow tract obstruction in the recipient
  - possibly coarctation of the aorta in the donor.
- Functional anomalies, even when severe, respond rapidly and, in many, completely following treatment.
- Acquired structural anomalies may progress both antenatally and postnatally even to the point of needing treatment.
- Thus postnatal cardiac assessments are appropriate to determine resolution or progression.
- Antenatally, both twins are subjected to risk factors for hypertension and thus postnatal blood pressure measurement is recommended.
- Changes in either twin may be fetal origins of adult disease (➔ Chapter 2).

Role of fetal echocardiography in monochorionic twin pregnancies

- There are well-defined protocols for timing of fetal medicine assessments but from the cardiac perspective.
- Detailed fetal cardiac anatomical assessment at 18–20 weeks.
- If normal and the pregnancy is uncomplicated, no further cardiac assessments are needed.
- If there is any suggestion of TTTS developing, cardiac assessment can refine Quintero staging.
- As a minimum, and as an achievable objective in a busy clinical practice, serial assessments of:
    - cardiac size
    - myocardial dimensions
    - subjective assessment of function
    - quantification of AV valve regurgitation
    - E/A ratios across AV valves
    - evidence of outflow tract obstruction
    - ductus venosus interrogation.

Chapter 24

The heart in the sick fetus

Introduction

- Separating maternal from fetal causes of fetal compromise is simplifying the reality of the closely integrated combined unit but serves as a method of classification, with much overlap.
- The fetus is vulnerable to changing environments including those brought about by some maternal diseases especially if maternal well-being is compromised.
- Major factors determining fetal cardiac output are discussed in other chapters (➔ Chapters 17 and 18) and include:
  - myocardial function, in particular right ventricular diastolic function
  - ventricular preload
  - ventricular afterload
  - heart rate.
- Assessment of both cardiovascular and biophysical profiles provide complementary information which can be monitored serially (➔ Chapter 17).
- Cardiac failure is the end-point reflecting inadequate tissue perfusion, acidosis, and tissue damage.
- Circulatory changes, sometimes involving fetal shunts, and including brain-sparing (➔ p. 273), aim to preserve function in more vital organs.

Maternal causes

Maternal diabetes

- The association with structural CHD is covered in ➲ Chapter 2.
- Fetal hyperinsulinaemia is associated with proliferation and hypertrophy of cardiac myocytes leading to cardiac hypertrophy (Fig. 24.1):
  - Particularly in the 3rd trimester.
  - Probably in proportion to the level of glycaemic control.
  - More often seen in macrosomic fetuses.
  - Rarely associated with fetal compromise.
  - May cause early neonatal symptoms/signs.
- Resolves spontaneously during first year of life.

Maternal anti-SSA/Ro antibodies

- Anti-SSA/Ro antibodies are usually present in women with connective tissue disorders including systemic lupus erythematosus and Sjögren syndrome.
- Disease in the fetus is unrelated to whether or not the mother has active disease.
- Many mothers are asymptomatic, the anti-Ro antibodies only being discovered during investigation of a fetus with heart block.
- The majority of fetuses with 'isolated' heart block (structurally normal hearts) are associated with maternal anti-Ro antibodies.
- Anti-Ro antibodies cross the placenta, mainly during the 2nd trimester, causing an immune-mediated inflammatory response in the fetal myocardium and AV conduction system, particularly affecting the AV node.

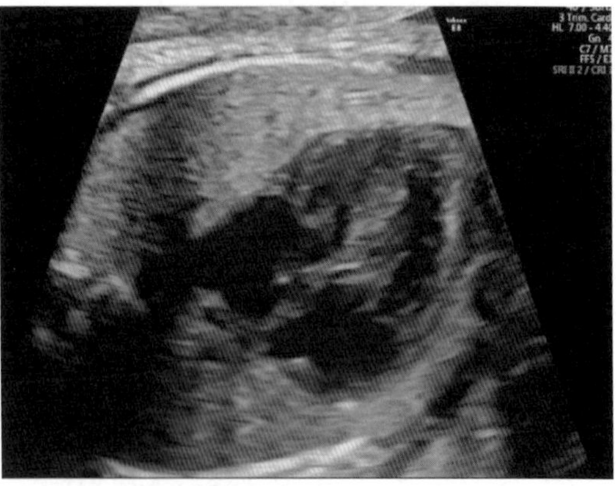

Fig. 24.1 4-chamber view showing IVS at least twice as thick as LV posterior wall and RV anterior wall in fetus of type 1 diabetic woman.

- This process may cause irreversible damage to the conducting tissue and lead to a degree of heart block (see Chapter 17):
  - 1st- and 2nd-degree block is not necessarily progressive and spontaneous resolution in the fetus has been documented.
- It may progress postnatally.
- 3rd-degree (complete) AV block is virtually always permanent.
- 2–3% of fetuses in mothers with anti-Ro antibodies develop complete heart block:
  - Recurrence in subsequent pregnancies increases to 20%.
- Rarely endocardial fibroelastosis may develop in any part of the heart:
  - With uncertain prognosis.
- Maternal medication with the aim of prevention is controversial and as yet unproven (➲ Chapter 17):
  - Maternal hydroxychloroquine possibly reduces the risk of heart block.
  - Maternal steroids are probably only indicated if there is evidence of an active inflammatory process, e.g. inappropriate pericardial fluid.
- If complete heart block develops, close monitoring of heart rate, function, and fetal well-being is appropriate.
- Ventricular rates above 50/min are usually well tolerated:
  - Presence of hydrops at an early stage suggests a guarded prognosis.
- In the presence of 2nd- or 3rd-degree heart block, delivery by caesarean section is usual as monitoring fetal well-being in labour is difficult.
- DCM may develop later in childhood.

Severe intrauterine growth restriction

- Placental dysfunction secondary to maternal factors can lead to increased placental vascular resistance.
- In the fetal circulation, up to 80% of the RV output returns directly to the placenta.
- Increased RV afterload may cause RV enlargement:
  - And a possible impact on systemic venous return to the RA.
  - These can be monitored as discussed in ➲ Chapter 18.
- Redistribution of flow to vital organs takes place including 'brain-sparing' involving redirection of flow at the aortic isthmus, cerebral vasodilation manifested as increased diastolic flow velocity.

Use of non-steroidal anti-inflammatory drugs

- See ➲ p. 254.

Maternal infections

- See ➲ Chapter 2.

Fetal causes

Structural congenital heart disease

- Most structural lesions are well tolerated in pregnancy.
- The few exceptions include:
  - Ebstein's anomaly/tricuspid valve dysplasia
  - critical aortic stenosis with a dilated LV
  - many cardiomyopathies
  - those in whom an arrhythmia is also present.
- See relevant chapters for further details.

Twin–twin transfusion syndrome

- Particularly in the recipient twin (➲ Chapter 23).

Fetal infection

- Infection is well recognized as a cause of fetal hydrops.
- Viral agents identified include adenoviruses and parvovirus.
- They may exert their effects either by:
  - inducing myocarditis
  - causing hepatitis and compromising protein production
  - by causing haemolytic anaemia (particularly parvovirus).

Premature closure of the ductus arteriosus

- The commonest recognized cause is the use of NSAIDs:
  - either specifically as an anti-tocolytic or to reduce liquor volume
  - or because of inadvertent maternal ingestion.
- Often no cause is identified though a careful drug, dietary, and complementary therapy history may reveal a possible aetiological factor.
- Narrowing or closure of the ductus arteriosus may be visible on 2D imaging:
  - usually in association with RV dilation.
- Colour and pulsed wave Doppler assessment demonstrate increased velocity both in systole and diastole (see Fig. 24.2a–c).
  - And thus a reduction in pulsatility index (PI) calculated from pulsed wave Doppler interrogation of the DA.
  - PI = systolic – diastolic velocities/mean velocity with normal range being 1.9–3 (Fig. 24.2d).
- Changes usually rapidly resolve if the precipitating factor is removed.
- Cardiac manifestations of a restricted DA include:
  - enlargement of the right heart (Fig. 24.3)
  - pulmonary artery
  - tricuspid regurgitation
  - pulmonary regurgitation
  - prominent pulmonary veins with increased pulmonary venous return.
- Indications for delivery are not clear cut but may include:
  - complete closure of the ductus arteriosus
  - severe and progressive tricuspid regurgitation

- progressive pulmonary regurgitation
- retrograde flow in the ductus venosus
- hydrops.
- Postnatally, there is a risk of pulmonary hypertension and right ventricular dysfunction.

Fetal anaemia

- May be caused by immune or non-immune factors.
- Haemodynamic changes include:
    - reduced oxygen-carrying capacity of the blood
    - increased cardiac output leading to a hyperdynamic circulation
    - increased middle cerebral artery systolic velocity, providing ventricular systolic function is not impaired.
- Middle cerebral artery Doppler velocity is a reliable tool for diagnosis.

Pleural effusions

- May be present in isolation—primary—or as part of a more general hydropic process (➔ Chapter 22).
- May be associated with other anomalies:
    - structural
    - syndromic
    - chromosomal
    - or with infections.
- Prognosis depends on size, gestation, whether uni- or bilateral, and the underlying aetiology, which is often unknown.
- Large effusions act as space-occupying lesions and may have a significant haemodynamic effect.
- Fetal intervention may have a dramatic effect but re-accumulation is common.

Fetal hydrops

- See ➔ Chapter 22.

Fetal cardiac arrhythmias

- See ➔ Chapter 17.

Fetal cardiomyopathies

- See ➔ Chapter 19.

Fetal arteriovenous fistulae

- Can occur in the liver, lung, coronary circulation, brain, placenta, or in conjunction with sacrococcygeal teratoma.
- May result in increased cardiac output.

Fetal cardiac tumours

- See ➔ Chapter 20.

(a)

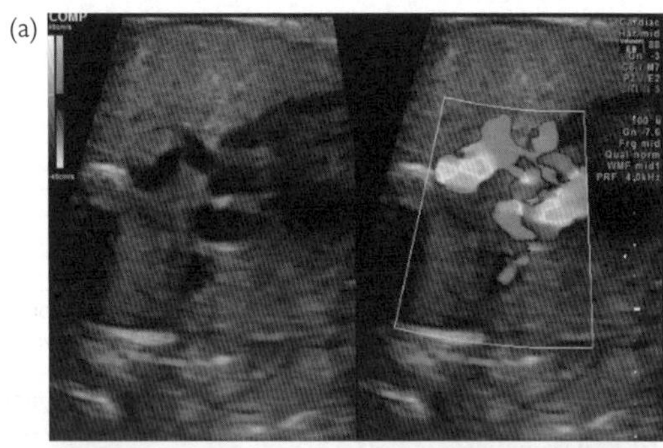

(b)

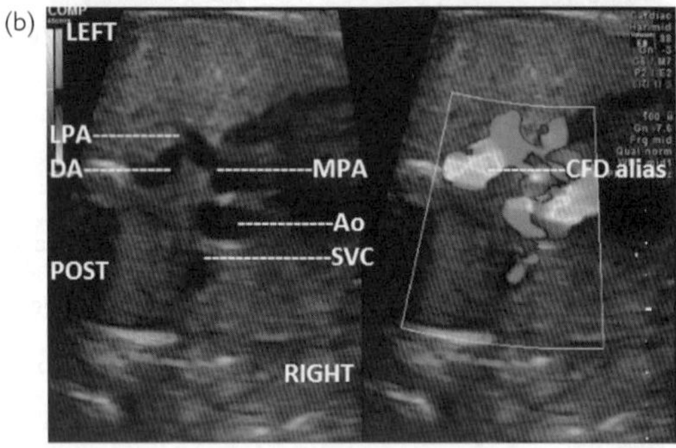

Fig. 24.2 Oblique 3-vessel view showing constriction at the PA end of the DA with increase in blood velocity across that region shown on colour flow Doppler. (See colour plate section). (a) (plain) and (b) (annotated). (c) Pulsed wave Doppler across constricted DA showing increase in systolic and diastolic velocity and low PI with DA constriction. (d) Chart of normal DA PI (systolic velocity – diastolic/mean velocity) used to evaluate and monitor DA constriction.

Part (d) adapted from Huhta JC (2005) Fetal congestive heart failure, *Seminars in Fetal & Neonatal Medicine* 10;542–52 with permission from Elsevier.

(c)

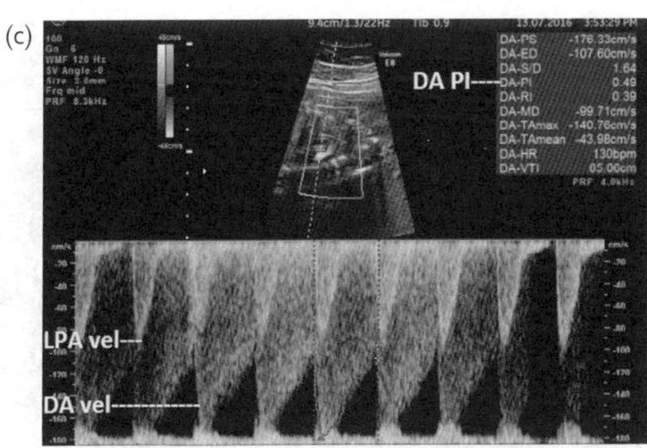

(d)

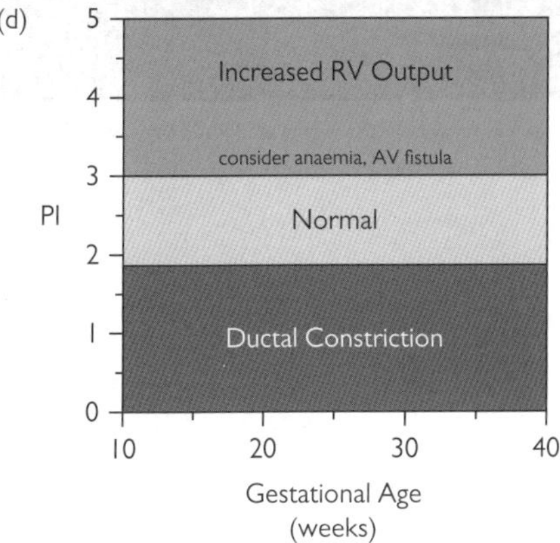

Fig. 24.2 (*Contd*)

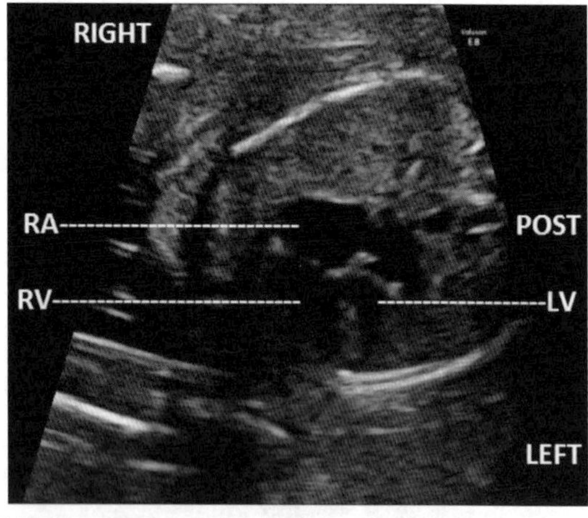

Fig. 24.3 4-chamber view in systole showing dilated RV in fetus with DA constriction.

Chapter 25

Pregnancy management of fetal cardiac disease

Introduction

- Cardiac abnormalities account for approximately 20% of neonatal deaths and in some the cardiac cause is only identified at postmortem.
- A falling proportion of CHD remains undetected during pregnancy.
- Many diagnoses only influence antenatal management with respect to communication and arranging postnatal cardiological review.
- There are some lesions for which prenatal diagnosis may improve postnatal outcome both in terms of mortality and morbidity.
- Most cardiac lesions do not alter pregnancy management and only very few are better delivered early or by elective caesarean section.
- A few lesions should be delivered where intervention is available on the same hospital campus such as:
  - simple transposition in case of the need for atrial septostomy
  - obstructed TAPVD (rarely diagnosed *in utero*)
  - possibly HLHS with obstructed foramen ovale if active management is intended, this is a matter for debate.
- Whether duct-dependent cardiac lesions are delivered in their local hospital or in a cardiac centre varies according to local facilities, expertise, and transport considerations as well as family preferences.
- After a diagnosis of CHD is made *in utero*, the aim is to optimize care for the fetus and the parents in pregnancy and in the newborn period.
- Some problems require close monitoring of the cardiac status during the pregnancy, e.g.:
  - tricuspid valve disease (➔ p. 112)
  - foramen ovale size in TGA and HLHS
  - lesions that may progress or regress as gestation advances
  - dysrhythmias
  - pericardial effusions
  - cardiac tumours
  - heart muscle disease.
- For other lesions, very little monitoring in pregnancy is required, such as isolated small or medium sized VSDs.
- In a very few cases, prenatal management might include some form of cardiac intervention during pregnancy, such as:
  - foramen ovale restricting flow in HLHS and TGA
  - optimizing ventricular growth in AS.
- Communication and updating of information with other members of the team—obstetrician, GP, midwife, and neonatologist in both the cardiac unit and local unit are crucial to integrated care.

Diagnosis

- Following the suspicion of a cardiac anomaly, prompt referral to a specialist unit is advisable where the diagnosis can be confirmed and explained.
- Involvement of a multidisciplinary team is appropriate so that non-cardiac problems including chromosomal, syndromic, and structural anomalies can be identified or, as far as is possible, excluded.
- This may also include discussion of the option for invasive testing.
- Important additional diagnostic information may be obtained as the pregnancy advances.

Counselling

- Following confirmation of a cardiac anomaly the family should be counselled in detail, including:
  - explanation of the cardiac diagnosis
  - possible postnatal management and treatment options
  - prognosis and guide to outcome for the cardiac diagnosis
  - likelihood for coexisting non-cardiac anomalies
  - potential for fetal compromise during the remainder of the pregnancy
  - clear diagrams and written notes for parents to take away for further reference are helpful
  - easy access route back for further discussion before the follow-up appointment if wanted.
- Figures for surgical outcome should be available for the unit involved as well as nationally (in UK available from the Central Cardiac Audit Database: http://www.ccad.org.uk/congenital) although this information requires a clear explanation and guidance as it may be difficult to interpret in the context of a prenatally diagnosed anomaly.
- It is important the family understands the following:
  - The limitations of prenatal diagnosis.
  - The concept of evolution of a cardiac lesion during pregnancy, usually with progression—particularly relevant if the anomaly is detected early in pregnancy.
  - The potential for the existence of further non-cardiac problems not identifiable prenatally which may significantly influence postnatal morbidity and mortality.
  - Limitations in knowledge such as long-term survival and quality of life following surgery for some lesions, including HLHS.
  - Cardiac anomalies identified prenatally tend towards the more severe end of the spectrum and are associated with higher morbidity and mortality before and after birth.
  - The possibility of termination when appropriate.
- Postnatal treatment options are now available for almost all forms of CHD, however severe; for some, treatment will be palliative with the possibility of several procedures before school age.
- Discussion should also include possible aetiologies; this may also provide an opportunity to reassure parents that the problem is unlikely to be due to factors within their control.
- Risk of intrauterine death is small but higher in presence of non-cardiac anomalies especially chromosomal or when associated with rhythm disturbances, particularly heart block.
- Termination of pregnancy is legal in the UK until 24 weeks; after that it is still possible if the abnormality is considered 'likely to cause serious handicap' but at the discretion of the obstetrician and this varies elsewhere.

- The possibility of providing compassionate care and no active treatment may also be included in discussion of situations where treatment is palliative with a high risk, as in the Norwood procedure for HLHS; however, as survival figures improve, this may cease to be an option.
- It is helpful if the referring clinician can prepare the family for the possibility of a problem; this allows them to arrange for both parents to attend.

As far as is possible, counselling should be non-directive and the family reassured that they have time to make important and far-reaching decisions; they need to know that whatever their choice they will be given support. They are likely to feel over-loaded with information and should be given the opportunity for further discussion on another occasion after they have had time to assimilate some of the facts. Advice as to which websites are helpful and accurate may also be appropriate; however, families should be encouraged to discuss any discrepancies they detect. (See 'Further reading'.)

Further reading

A selection of useful websites includes:
British Heart Foundation: www.bhf.org.uk
Boston Children's Hospital: www.childrenshospital.org
Royal Children's Hospital Melbourne: www.rch.org.au/cardiology/parent info/parent information

Management of the pregnancy

- The presence of a cardiac anomaly diagnosed prenatally does not usually need to influence management of the pregnancy.
- For the few cardiac lesions where early delivery is a possibility, administration of maternal steroids may be appropriate in order to aid maturity of the fetal lungs.
- Meanwhile, fetal well-being should be monitored in the usual way.
- For pregnancies where delivery in the local unit is planned, a reliable method of alerting the neonatologist to the forthcoming birth is essential, along with guidelines as to what early postnatal management is appropriate and when and who should be contacted after delivery.
- For pregnancies where delivery is planned in a unit with cardiac facilities, it is still important to ensure the local team have clear guidelines for perinatal care in case delivery takes place locally.
- For cardiac lesions where progression is recognized to be a significant risk, regular (monthly, reducing the interval to 2-weekly near term) assessments can help to determine optimal time and place for delivery.
- The likelihood for duct dependency may become apparent during serial monitoring in cases where progression of the lesion can be demonstrated.
- Intrauterine death in the presence of CHD is unusual; factors increasing the risk of IUD include
  - presence of karyotypic anomalies
  - presence of extracardiac structural anomalies
  - structural CHD associated with complete heart block
  - few specific cardiac lesions including tricuspid dysplasia, Ebstein's anomaly, and critical aortic stenosis.
- Prematurity (delivery before 36 weeks) significantly increases morbidity and mortality in babies born with severe CHD, especially in the presence of non-cardiac anomalies.
- For management of arrhythmias, see ➔ Chapter 17.
- Some families wish to meet the surgeon before delivery; many value the opportunity to meet with cardiac liaison nurses at some point.
- Induction labour may be appropriate if delivery in the cardiac centre is planned.

Fetal intervention

- Fetal treatment of cardiac arrhythmias is well established as effective (➲ Chapter 17).
- The benefit of fetal intervention for structural cardiac anomalies is widely debated.
- Safety of the mother is the first priority.

Catheter intervention has been performed for several cardiac lesions including:

- Aortic stenosis and pulmonary stenosis:
  - The stimulus for growth of chambers and vessels is blood flow.
  - In the presence of significant stenosis of a valve, blood may take an alternative route of lower resistance resulting in further valvar obstruction or chamber underdevelopment.
  - It is usually assumed that to have 2 functioning ventricles—a 'biventricular circulation'—postnatally is preferable to a palliated single-ventricle circulation.
  - The objective for offering *in utero* balloon valvuloplasty for aortic or pulmonary stenosis is to maintain flow through the stenotic valve and to encourage growth of the corresponding chambers with the aim of achieving a biventricular circulation postnatally.
- Hypoplastic left heart syndrome:
  - In HLHS, unrestricted flow through the atrial septum is essential for survival *in utero* and immediately postnatally.
  - In HLHS, there is potential for the atrial septum to close; this can lead to hydrops and intrauterine death
  - Performing an atrial septostomy *in utero* may be achievable but the gap created tends to close soon afterwards; insertion of a stent in the atrial septum may allow patency to be preserved.
  - It is unclear as to whether or not this has postnatal benefit in terms of less diseased pulmonary vasculature.

Such invasive techniques carry with them a risk of inducing miscarriage or preterm labour as well as a small risk of haemorrhage, infection, and intrauterine death. These procedures are technically challenging, and involve teamwork and collaboration between fetal medicine specialists and cardiologists. Concentration of treatments in a few centres and careful documentation of cases are likely to give the best results and reliable data on efficacy.

Management of delivery

- Timing and method of delivery does not usually need to be altered in the presence of a cardiac anomaly; the normal obstetric indications for instrumental delivery or caesarean section should be followed.
- Where significant distances may be involved, induction near term may be appropriate to avoid travelling in labour if delivery in the cardiac centre is planned.
- Most fetuses with CHD tolerate labour well although exceptions to this would include:
  - sustained arrhythmias in whom monitoring of fetal well-being during labour would be impossible
  - fetuses with compromised cardiac function and a low cardiovascular profile score
  - fetal hydrops.

Place of delivery

- Place of delivery may be influenced by a number of factors including diagnosis, local resources, and parental preference; if delivery is likely to be by caesarean section, prenatal transfer to a cardiac unit minimizes the risk of separation if a neonatal procedure is required.
- Different cardiac units have their own policies for where babies known to have CHD should ideally be delivered and have a working relationship with their referring neonatal departments.
- If very early intervention is anticipated, as when the atrial septum is restrictive in HLHS or TGA (see ➔ Chapters 10 and 13), delivery should be where an early atrial septostomy can be performed.
- For duct-dependent lesions (see Table 25.1) the policy will be different in various units but many neonatal units are able to start prostaglandin and discuss further management with the paediatric cardiac service.

Table 25.1 Duct-dependent cardiac lesions

Left sided	Right sided	Mixed
Critical aortic stenosis	Critical pulmonary stenosis	Transposition*
Aortic atresia	Pulmonary atresia with intact ventricular septum	
Hypoplastic left heart syndrome	Pulmonary atresia with VSD (including severe tetralogy of Fallot)*	
Coarctation of the aorta*	Tricuspid atresia*	
Interrupted aortic arch		

* Not all are duct dependent.

Future pregnancies

Following a pregnancy with CHD—whether with a successful outcome or resulting in termination of pregnancy or intrauterine death—an opportunity must be given to discuss all aspects including:

- risks to future pregnancies
- any specific preconception measures (e.g. changing drug management of maternal disease)
- the nature and timing of relevant fetal assessments and diagnostic procedures in future pregnancies.

Chapter 26

Neurodevelopment and fetal cardiac disease

Introduction

The potential for cerebral perfusion to be compromised in a fetus with structural or functional heart disease is an important but as yet poorly understood issue.

Counselling for a fetal structural cardiac lesion includes discussion of possible additional non-cardiac problems for which the cardiac lesion may serve as a marker and which may themselves have a greater impact on survival and quality of life than the cardiac lesion itself. There is increasing interest as to whether this discussion should include the unquantified association between CHD and potential for compromised neurodevelopment; in practice, it is not uncommon for parents to raise this question themselves.

- Many studies are in progress to try to address this problem.
- Different methods are used to try to quantify the impact of altered haemodynamics on cerebral perfusion in the vulnerable fetal brain.
- Evaluation of neurodevelopment in neonates and beyond in clinical practice is not always straightforward, particularly if they are acutely or chronically unwell.
- Evaluation is complicated and separating fetal factors from early infancy factors remains a challenge:
    - Especially in those having major cardiac surgery in the first few days of life.
    - And in those with other factors including prematurity and genetic syndromes.
    - If the risk of neurodevelopmental delay is overstated, termination of pregnancy may be requested because of this fear, even though expectations would be good for the cardiac diagnosis alone.

Haemodynamics

- The fetal circulation allows the most highly oxygenated arterial blood to be directed to the brain and myocardium as the ductus venosus directs highly oxygenated blood from the placenta into the RA, across the atrial septum to the LA to LV and ascending aorta.
- Normal fetal cerebral blood oxygen saturation is approximately 75%.
- Alteration of these blood flow patterns may reduce the supply to myocardium and brain of:
  - oxygen
  - glucose and other metabolic substrates.
- Oxygen saturation in the cerebral arterial blood has been found to be reduced in certain forms of structural CHD:
  - 50% in HLHS
  - 43% in TGA.
- The ductus arteriosus directs less highly oxygenated blood from the systemic veins to the RA, to the RV, to the PA, and then into the descending aorta to return to the placenta.

Specific cardiac lesions

The concern is mainly with:

- Lesions where cerebral perfusion is retrograde via the arterial duct, e.g. critical aortic stenosis and HLHS:
  - Cerebral blood flow may be reduced and will have lower oxygen levels than normal.
- Lesions with altered streaming, e.g. TGA:
  - Blood from the placenta and via ductus venosus is directed across the atrial septum to the LA, to the LV, and then to the lungs via the PA.
  - Blood from the RV with lower oxygen saturation (and possibly glucose content as well) thus perfuses the coronary and cerebral vessels.
- Possibly in lesions with increased mixing, e.g. tetralogy of Fallot.
- Possibly in association with poor function and hydrops, from whatever cause including arrhythmias.

Methods of assessment

Several different methods are used, all relatively crude, to establish and quantify alterations in cerebral perfusion and associated development and include the following.

Assessment of cerebral blood flow redistribution

- Using PW Doppler to measure MCA PI to detect evidence of cerebral vasodilation (i.e. attempting 'brain sparing').
- Brain sparing describes the process of cerebral redistribution to improve oxygen delivery to the brain.
- A reduction in MCA PI, similar to that seen in fetal hypoxia with growth restriction, has been demonstrated in fetuses with HLHS, progressively in the 3rd trimester.
- In some studies, cerebral vasodilatation was associated with better neurodevelopmental outcome; in others, a worse outcome.
- It is not clear if cerebral vasodilation detected in this way correlates with neurodevelopmental outcome.

Assessment of brain weight and volume

- Using MRI.
- *In utero* ± neonatally to estimate global brain volumes.
- In some studies, 3rd-trimester fetuses with certain forms of CHD have smaller total brain volumes than weight-adjusted fetuses with normal hearts.
- The relationship between brain size and function is complex.
- Other studies have found that antenatally detected brain abnormalities are relatively mild and thus their predictive value is unknown.
- Thus the correlation of MRI findings and neuropathology remains inconclusive.

Neurodevelopmental testing in childhood

- Standard testing throughout school years and includes:
  - Cognition
  - Motor skills
  - Communication skills
  - Daily living and adaptive behaviour.
- Any deviation from the norm can be the result of many genetic, congenital, and acquired factors.

Prevention or damage limitation

All theoretical at present but include:

- fetal intervention:
    - e.g. aortic balloon valvuloplasty in critical aortic stenosis to encourage forward flow around the aortic arch
- maternal hyperoxygenation:
    - fetal brain size has been correlated with fetal ascending aorta oxygen saturation and cerebral oxygen consumption.

Parental counselling

The impact of CHD in the fetus on cerebral development is difficult to quantify:

- It is important not to overstate the potential impact, as the evidence is still unclear.
- However, it is appropriate to discuss the dilemma for certain lesions.

Chapter 27

Postnatal evaluation

Introduction

There are differences between fetal and postnatal investigations for a variety of reasons. Members of the fetal team need to be aware of the scope of post-delivery tests so that prenatal management including counselling is consistent with later approaches. Ways in which tests are similar or differ post delivery are outlined in the following topics.

History and examination

- Both cardiac and non-cardiac diagnoses may be modified by post-delivery assessment, in particular some syndrome diagnoses may be more obvious.
- Re-evaluation of parental and family history may be indicated if previously unsuspected syndromal diagnoses need to be considered and investigated.
- If a cardiac or non-cardiac abnormality is suspected postnatally which was thought to have been excluded by fetal evaluation, it is important to reinvestigate.
- Cardiac conditions not usually detected *in utero* which may have syndromic implications include:
    - William's syndrome (pulmonary artery branch stenosis, supravalvar aortic stenosis)
    - Holt–Oram syndrome (ASD).; autosomal dominant
    - Wolff–Parkinson–White syndrome (short PR interval on ECG), occasionally familial
    - Alagille syndrome (pulmonary artery branch stenoses)
    - many cardiomyopathies with genetic and/or metabolic causes.

Echocardiography

A cardiac diagnosis made before delivery should be confirmed by echocardiography in live-born infants. The timing of this assessment will depend on the abnormality and a plan should be clearly stated in fetal reports in maternal case notes. Any discrepancy between fetal cardiac diagnosis and neonatal clinical assessment should be investigated as indicated by the clinical picture.

Radiology

Chest X-ray, computed tomography angiography, and cardiac angiography (cardiac catheterization) are all used in the evaluation of infants with cardiac disease. In some cases this can be predicted antenatally, allowing parents to be informed of the likely postnatal course of events. Interventional cardiac catheterization is used to treat a number of conditions (e.g. pulmonary atresia or critical pulmonary stenosis) and is done under X-ray control. Balloon atrial septostomy (most usually for TGA) is often done using ultrasound guidance.

Magnetic resonance imaging

This is widely used in evaluation of CHD in infants and children whereas it is not clinically used often in the fetus because of the problems of movement and of ECG gating. It does require heavy sedation or more often general anaesthesia in the infant and therefore is less used than computed tomography scanning which does not usually require anaesthesia. In the evaluation of some pathologies, postmortem MRI is considered; this is not particularly valuable in structural heart disease.

Electrocardiography

Is used postnatally for:

- determining cardiac rhythm
- assessing risk of arrhythmia (e.g. short PR, long QT interval)
- assessing heart muscle disease
- assessing structural heart disease.

Chromosome analysis and gene testing

- In live born or dead fetuses, blood lymphocytes, skin fibroblasts (easily obtained if cardiac surgical intervention planned), and other tissue can be obtained for analysis if prenatal samples are not available.
- Cord blood sampling may be valuable in making/confirming genetic diagnoses; this requires careful planning and good communication.
- Additional diagnoses may be entertained and warrant further testing of previously obtained samples.
- Tissue should be stored for later analysis if diagnostic doubt exists.
- Samples from other family members are becoming increasingly relevant, this requires sensitive counselling.
- See ➲ Chapter 8 for details of these tests.

Metabolic testing

The following should be borne in mind:

- Storage disorders associated with cardiac hypertrophy may not be recognized on fetal echocardiography.
- Fetal echocardiography has a low sensitivity and specificity for many metabolic conditions with myocardial involvement.
- If a precise diagnosis can be made on biochemical grounds, this usually requires postnatal investigation.
- Enzyme deficiencies or known gene defects may be detectable by invasive prenatal as well as by postnatal testing but samples usually take a considerable time to process.
- If a metabolic disorder is suspected prenatally, the fetal team needs to ensure the appropriate post-delivery investigations are planned beforehand whenever possible.
- Specialist advice is needed in order to investigate and manage suspected metabolic disorders efficiently.

Autopsy examination

No matter at what stage and under what circumstances death occurs, autopsy examination is highly desirable for the following reasons:

- To confirm, refute, or modify any diagnoses made both for the sake of the family and of the professionals involved.
- To allow as accurate a prediction as possible to be made about the risk of recurrence and the relevance of a diagnosis to other family members.
- Full autopsy may not be possible or consented to, but the following aspects need to be considered:
    - Gross anatomy of all systems.
    - Histology of definitely or possibly abnormal tissues.
    - Chromosomal and genetic sampling.
    - Imaging (e.g. bone X-rays, brain MRI).
    - Biochemical/metabolic sampling.
    - Storage of DNA for later testing.

It is most helpful to have a lead clinician who coordinates results and communicates with the family. It is important for this person to identify unanswered questions and to ensure a mechanism is in place for dealing with these in the future in the light of new medical or family information.

Index

D

E

F

G

H

I